re cov er

FINDING FREEDOM
WITH FOOD AGAIN

SUNNY YINGLING, MS, RD, CSSD

First edition: January 2020

Book design by Chris Hensley

Edited by Affordable Editing Services (www.affordableeditingservices.com)

ISBN 978-1-7332952-0-8 (paperback)

ISBN 978-1-7332952-1-5 (ebook)

Published by Sunny Yingling, MS, RD, CSSD

syingling@planhealthfitness.com

www.therecoverbook.com

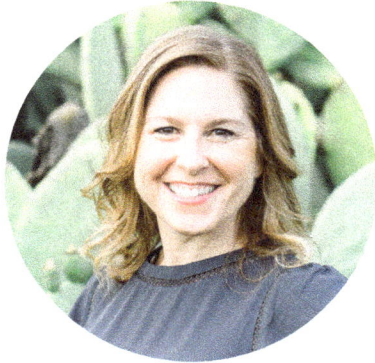

ABOUT THE AUTHOR

Sunny is a registered dietitian and Director of Nutrition with Plan Health & Fitness in Fresno, California. She earned her bachelor's degree from Biola University in physical education and earned her master's degree in nutrition science at San Jose State University. Sunny then returned to her home town to complete her dietetic internship with CSU Fresno. Her graduate research focused on the effects of fish oil supplements on cardiovascular disease risk; this research was presented at the annual meetings of both the California Dietetic Association and American Dietetic Association in 2008.

Sunny has been providing outpatient nutrition counseling since becoming a dietitian, and specializes in eating disorders, sports nutrition, and weight management. She also taught nutrition at Clovis Community College Center for several years and was the dietitian for the former Summit Eating Disorder and Outreach Program's intensive outpatient program. She is a Board Certified Specialist in Sports Dietetics with the Commission on Dietetic Registration and enjoys serving the needs of high school, collegiate, and recreational athletes. Sunny has provided nutrition education through presentations to varying audiences across the Central Valley and has made many public appearances for local media. Sunny is also a published writer for various websites and you can find her blog posts at www.planhealthfitness.com/bulletin/.

Sunny lives with her awesome husband and 3 very active children in Clovis, California and appreciates being able to serve the community she grew up in. She is thankful to be in private practice where she gets to balance family and work life. She has helped lead Plan Health and Fitness' run club for several years and you can often find her family out on the running trails. Sunny grew up with a passion for sports and recreation and loves that she gets to incorporate these interests into her professional pursuits. Growing up in the sport of gymnastics, Sunny had early exposure to unhealthy talk about food and weight and has heard the messages you may have heard throughout life. However, as she progressed in her nutrition education and continuing education to this day, she experiences freedom in her food choices, loves to eat, loves to cook, and loves to build experiences with others around food. You can find her on social media including Instagram @sunnyyingling or #mysunnystylediet.

ACKNOWLEDGEMENTS

I have to start by thanking my husband, Adam. From encouraging me when I decided to write a book in our crazy season of life, to reading every line and every chapter numerous times, to managing our kids while I wrote at coffee shops…..I couldn't have done this without your amazing support. You are truly the best teammate in my life.

Thank you to the friends and family that prayed for me and supported me, even by the simple act of asking how the writing was going. I felt surrounded by so much strength.

Thank you to my clients who were willing to jump in and provide their favorite recipes. I appreciate each of you for your time, your effort, and your belief in this book. It's my sincerest hope that you find freedom in your eating each and every day.

Thank you to the professional support around me from people who are great at what they do: Larry and Roberta Wennik at Affordable Editing Services, you kept me moving and taught me so much through this process. Chris Hensley, you have an amazing and creative mind. Danielle Wraith, you have such a gift behind the camera. And to the dietitians who brainstormed with me, encouraged me, and especially to those who reviewed the book in detail. What an incredible team!

Thank you to my God and Savior, you are my Rock. I can accomplish all things with you. Thank you for holding my hand when I need it most.

TABLE OF CONTENTS

INTRODUCTION

"Dieting is based on the misconception that food has a moral value. You probably have heard someone say something like, 'I've been good all day. Now I'm going to be bad and eat a slice of pumpkin pie.' But eating pie is not a 'bad' thing to do. Food does NOT have a moral value. Food is just food."

Jenni Schaefer

Author of Life Without ED (ED stands for Eating Disorder)

This quote from Jenni Schaefer is one of my favorites. It puts food into perspective—it's meant for nourishing, fueling, and protecting our bodies, and providing pleasure. And yet, in our diet-saturated culture, food has become a source of fear and guilt. If your ability to enjoy all foods is disrupted by fear; if you label foods as "good" and "bad", if eating from your personal "do not eat" list leaves you feeling anxious and ashamed, this book is for you. I often have clients that feel the need to compensate for "naughty" behavior after eating anything on their "bad" list, such as restricting calories the next day or compulsively taking off to the gym. But if you can transition from labeling these foods as "bad" to labeling them as "delicious and satisfying," there is nothing to compensate for. You simply enjoyed your meal or snack.

It's time to stop evaluating your worth by whether you did or didn't eat a cookie. Too often I hear conversations between people bragging about what foods they avoid. "I NEVER eat processed foods." "I would NEVER eat fast food." And somehow, it's embraced as a sign of good character. These "NEVER" statements simply lead to more limited food options and feelings of deprivation.

I was once eating at an Italian restaurant, and the waiter found out I was a dietitian. That night, I really wanted spaghetti and meatballs (I take great pleasure in a tasty meatball!). The waiter questioned my meal decision and was nearly trying to argue me out of the decision, "Are you SURE that's what you want? I thought you said you were a dietitian." He seemed to imply that I was abandoning my values as an RD by ordering a meatball. Maybe if I ordered a salad he would've felt more at ease.

I invite you to learn about the nutritional value of different foods, to dispel all the crazy myths surrounding foods, food groups (such as grains and dairy), and nutrients (such as carbs and fats). I invite you to begin adding a variety of foods back into your diet and refresh your palate. I don't want you to take food to social events in fear that you won't be able to eat anything prepared by the host. Each chapter will present sound evidence and build a case for both why and how you can incorporate different foods into your diet. My hope is that you will transition from labeling foods as "good" or "bad" or simply as a caloric number. Instead, you'll be able to include foods based on how they can benefit your body, your mind, and your spirit.

In Chapter 1, you'll start by revisiting the word, "calories," a word that's been vilified in our culture. You'll focus on food as a source of fuel and much needed energy, providing you with a life full of vitality and strength. Continuing with a focus on energy, in Chapter 2 you'll read about carbohydrates. I'll discuss the specific sources of carbohydrates that are rich sources of nutrients and components of a healthy digestive system. In Chapter 3, you'll not only learn about the nutritional benefits of fats, but their function in providing flavor (and enjoyment!) in your foods. Chapter 4 is about protein, the building block of your body. A specific emphasis is placed on understanding meat and dairy products as they relate to your health.

In Chapter 5, you'll learn how to fit sweets and desserts into your diet. I'll discuss the importance of pleasure and satisfaction in your eating experiences and will challenge the myths surrounding added sugars. In Chapter 6, you'll read about eating at restaurants, with specific tips on how to choose menu items, how to reduce guilt and anxiety associated with eating out, and how to find delight in the dining-out experience. You'll notice, Chapters 5 and 6 delve deeper into disordered behaviors, since desserts and dining out are two of the greatest challenges for many of my clients. Finally, in Chapter 7, I finish with a focus on exercise as medicine. Instead of exercise being solely used as a method of weight loss, I'll discuss alternate benefits to exercise and help you create your own exercise plan. (This is assuming it is medically appropriate that you engage in regular exercise.)

Each of chapters 1-5 concludes with a list of recipes for you that were contributed by my past and current eating disorder clients. Some of them wanted to share their comments with you as encouragement for tasting their dishes. These people have been, and some still are, in the fight for freedom from "fear of foods". However, they've achieved so much by learning what you will read about in this book. Use this book as a tool along your journey as you *recover* from eating with anxiety and fear.

1

THE FOCUS ON FOOD AS ENERGY

CALORIES

How is it that the word "calories" has such a negative connotation? We are bombarded with messages that tell us to minimize our calories, watch our calories, and control our calories—messages from social media, news, family, peers, and even doctors and health educators—as many of my clients will testify. It may not help that recent legislation and food labeling changes promote a focus on calories. All restaurants and retail food establishments with at least 20 locations are required to provide calorie information for all food and beverage items. Additionally, upcoming changes to the Nutrition Facts Panel on food and beverage product packaging includes the word "Calories" in larger print. This makes calories more easily identifiable, drawing greater attention to the word. With the current high obesity rate in the U.S., a focus on calories is unlikely to diminish. When you note calories on packaging, in restaurants, and online, my goal is for you to shift from fearing the number to appreciating that this number represents the energy for your body to run on.

REVISITING THE WORD CALORIES

What are calories? According to Mosby's Medical Dictionary (and other scientific resources), a calorie is:

- The amount of heat needed to raise the temperature of 1 kilogram of water 1°C

- A unit, equal to the large calorie, used to denote the heat expenditure of an organism and the fuel or energy value of food.

Did you catch those words in the second definition? A unit that describes the ENERGY VALUE of food. One of the characteristics of foods and beverages is that they provide you with energy!

If you need help changing your mindset about calories, try substituting the word "energy" each time you evaluate calories in foods and beverages. Create a positive visual of how that food will promote the energy you need, such as the delivery of nutrients to your brain and central nervous system. I have numerous clients who complain of feeling sluggish. They meet with me to explore ways of achieving more energy. According to a 2011 study reported by the Centers for Disease Control and Prevention (CDC), approximately 15% of women and 10% of men complained of "feeling very tired or exhausted" over a 3-month period.

Additionally, an article released by the Washington Post in 2017 indicated that about 5 million medical visits each year are attributed to complaints of fatigue. Unfortunately, we've seen an increase in the use of stimulants, such as energy drinks, evidence that people are seeking to address this issue on their own. Would it surprise you to know that, in 2016, the energy drink market worldwide was a 43-billion-dollar industry? According to market research in 2017, this industry is expected to continue to increase until 2025. Researchers stated, "Almost 60% of the male and 40% of the female population in the U.S. is addicted to these beverages." My hope is that you don't rely on any supplemental stimulant. One of the important keys to overall energy is eating and drinking ENOUGH calories. Period.

Your body works hard capturing the energy you consume through foods and beverages. Calories are essential. They are good for you and not something to avoid. There is a nutrition concept called *physiological fuel value*. This is the difference between the number of calories from food (measured in a laboratory) and what your body actually digests and absorbs for energy. Your body is not 100% efficient at using every calorie you consume. To overcome some of the challenges in your digestive system and improve efficiency, there are many mechanisms in place in your gastrointestinal (GI) tract.

CAPTURING CALORIES

The goal of digestion is to break down large pieces of food into smaller components that can be absorbed in the GI tract. This process starts in the mouth, using a digestive enzyme called *amylase*, which begins breaking down carbohydrates. The simple act of chewing mechanically breaks food down into smaller pieces, allowing you to swallow the food more easily and for the food to move down the GI tract more efficiently. Once food enters the stomach, there are digestive juices that continue the process of breaking down the food. The

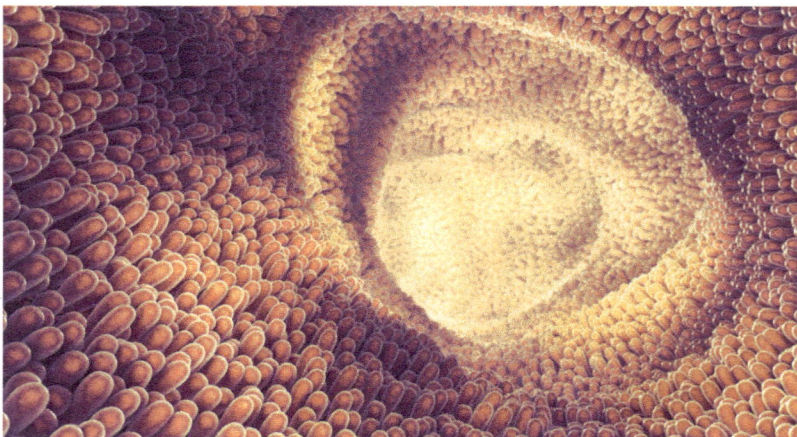

Villi and microvilli of the small intestine

stomach is an extremely acidic environment, which promotes the breakdown of proteins. Finally, the small intestine is where digestion is completed and most of the absorption of nutrients occurs. It measures about 7 meters or about 21 feet in length. That length provides a greater opportunity for absorption to take place. Additionally, the small intestine has finger-like projections, called "villi", with even smaller hair-like projections called "microvilli". They further help increase the surface area of the small intestine by over 600 times! The more surface area means more opportunity for digestion and absorption of nutrients.

Another way your body works to capture energy and nutrients is by adapting how quickly or slowly food moves through the GI tract. Many of my clients who are severely undereating complain of nausea, bloating, and constipation. These symptoms are related to the slowing of the movement of food through the tract. This is the body's way of compensating for fewer calories. The longer food sits in the GI tract, the more time there is for absorption of calories and nutrients. The body maximizes the opportunity for obtaining energy from food because of the limited amount of food my clients are eating. Again, this contributes to unwanted GI issues.

Bottom line: Calories are important for your life—they are **not** the enemy of your health.

CONSEQUENCES OF STARVATION AND DIETING

Fatigue. Exhaustion. Weakness. Lethargy. As mentioned earlier, one of the first consequences of consuming too few calories is low energy. When dietitians assess energy needs of a person, the first part of the analysis is to identify someone's basal metabolic rate (BMR). This is the energy required to support the basic functions of the body to sustain life. For example, it's the energy used by the lungs as you inhale and exhale, by the heart to pump blood, and by the kidneys as they filter out waste and fluids. It's the energy used to keep you warm and maintain body temperature, and it's the energy required by your brain to send signals throughout the body. (Your brain uses more energy than any other bodily organ!) BMR is measured when someone is both physically and mentally at rest.

If you significantly restrict your calorie intake, you're decreasing your BMR as your body slows down in response to the low energy. It is a protective mechanism by the body as it adapts to preserve your vital functions. A 2015 study reported that consuming only 50% of caloric needs for 3 weeks leads to an average reduction of 266 calories burned each day by study subjects. A slower metabolism means less calories burned. If you were trying to lose weight by restricting your calories, you actually encouraged your metabolism to slow down. You likely made your weight goals harder to reach.

Additionally, there seems to be a linear relationship between the drop in metabolic rate and the reduction of calories. For example, if a sedentary person eats 70% of 1200 calories a day for at least 2 months, that person's metabolic rate is expected to decrease to 70% of normal. Again, fewer calories means slower metabolism. Along with the slower metabolic rate comes a decrease in body temperature. Picture your metabolic rate as a fire in your body's core. Without enough fuel for the fire, the flame diminishes in order to preserve essential functions of the body. With prolonged starvation, those essential functions slowly decline. A common question I get from clients is how to support a healthy or strong metabolism. My basic response is always, "Start by eating enough." Low energy in leads to low energy out.

THE HEART

The effect starvation has on the heart is particularly concerning. In the absence of adequate nutrition, the body will use skeletal muscle to provide energy. The heart muscle, therefore, is broken down as fuel for the body, leading to a weaker heart muscle and the possibility of future heart failure. A low heart-rate and low blood-pressure can be indicative of damage to the heart muscle. If you are an athlete with a low heart-rate accompanied by low caloric intake, don't assume the low heart-rate is simply due to your high fitness level. The heart can become deconditioned, which is evidenced by a large jump in heart-rate while doing a simple task like brushing your teeth.

THE INTESTINES

As mentioned above, other consequences of starvation are GI issues, especially constipation. This is a common complaint for those consuming very few calories, whether from dieting or engaging in restricting behaviors. Because of the low volume of food, the body has much less to get rid of. There's simply not enough for the body to push through the GI tract. Because the movement of the food is slowed down, the food remains longer without being eliminated.

Longer-term starvation can weaken the muscles of the GI tract, leaving them too feeble for the job of pushing the contents of your food through the tube. Consider the effect of lifting weights on your bicep muscles. With consistency and adequate weight, performing bicep curls leads to strength and the ability to continue optimal function. You are providing work for the muscle to perform. The muscles of your GI tract behave the same way; you must provide work for them in order to keep them strong and operating optimally. That work is provided in the form of an appropriate amount of food.

THE BRAIN

As we think about our organs, it's easy to miss the essential provision of energy to the brain. Starvation will hinder vital neurological functions by starving the brain. Clients often complain of difficulty focusing and concentrating because thoughts about food interfere with normal functioning. As I perform assessments with new clients, I ask, "How much time do you spend thinking about food?" Those with disordered eating behaviors respond that their thoughts not only interfere during the day, but interrupt sleep patterns and permeate their dreams. The brain is literally "screaming" for energy.

Starvation and dieting promote irritability and encourage mood disorders. Clinical research supports a strong association between malnutrition / starvation and anxiety / depression. Though not completely understood at this time, the relationship may be due to a reduction in the activity of serotonin, a neurotransmitter or chemical messenger between nerve cells. Serotonin promotes feelings of happiness and overall well-being. Irritability is a common side-effect that is partially due to the feeling of unsatisfied hunger. You may be familiar with the phrase "hangry," which is used to describe a state of feeling angry due to hunger. Those that recognize the relationship between irritability and hunger can respond appropriately by eating to calm their mood. However, with prolonged starvation, the hunger cues are silenced and many of my clients no longer connect hunger to feelings of irritability.

THE BODY TISSUES

Finally, starvation and dieting may result in physical consequences that affect appearance, especially with prolonged starvation. Common symptoms include dry brittle nails, thinning or loss of hair, dry skin, and loss of fat pads under the eyes. The body doesn't have enough energy, fat, and protein to support healthy maintenance of these tissues. Moreover, there is a rare digestive disorder called superior mesenteric artery syndrome that results from the loss of the fat pad around an artery in your midsection. The first part of the small intestine becomes compressed between two arteries because of the loss of this fat pad. And this leads to GI issues, including vomiting, nausea, and pain. While this is a rare complication, the mechanism is the same—inadequate energy compromises the body's ability to maintain important tissues.

While this section does not provide an exhaustive list of consequences, I want you to understand what may happen with dieting and starvation. Too often, a low-calorie intake is glorified in our culture as a way to lose weight, without an adequate understanding of possible unwanted results.

THE FEMALE ATHLETE TRIAD AND RED-S

The female athlete triad describes the relationship between low energy availability, menstrual dysfunction (e.g., amenorrhea) and low bone-mineral density (osteoporosis).

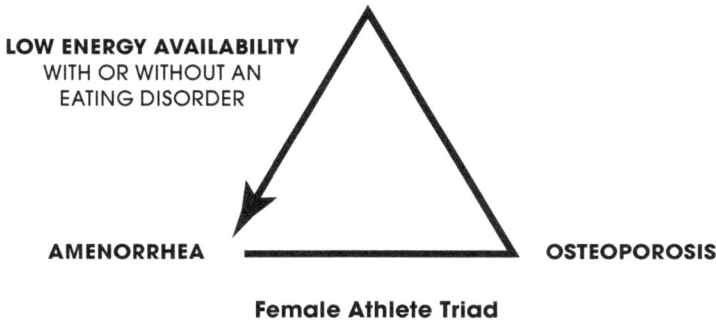

LOW ENERGY AVAILABILITY
WITH OR WITHOUT AN
EATING DISORDER

AMENORRHEA　　　　　　　　**OSTEOPOROSIS**

Female Athlete Triad

According to the American College of Sports Medicine, energy availability is defined as "dietary energy intake minus exercise energy expenditure." It's the energy left over for other physiological functions after accounting for the calories used during exercise. It also includes requirements for growth and menstruation. Inadequate energy forces the body to compromise these processes. Low energy availability may result from intentionally restricting calories or from increasing exercise. In either case, the potential consequences are the same. In recent years, the term "relative energy deficiency in sport" (RED-S) has been established. This syndrome takes a more comprehensive approach and identifies the consequences of low energy availability beyond menstrual dysfunction and bone health. It recognizes that energy deficiency impairs the function of other organs, may lead to psychological issues, and affects male athletes, as well.

Menstrual dysfunction includes both oligomenorrhea (greater than 35 days between menstrual cycles) and amenorrhea (an absence of cycles for at least 3 months). While many women may decide that the absence of a menstrual period as desirable (not feeling encumbered by bleeding every month and/or being concerned with iron losses), amenorrhea is associated with significant potential problems. Foremost is the issue of infertility (due to the inability to ovulate) and disrupted luteal function. In females, a surge of luteinizing hormone (LH) is responsible for ovulation. From my experience with clients, the ability to have children may be the only motivating factor to promote adequate energy intake. If this is you, it may be a good place to start. Becoming pregnant and maintaining a healthy pregnancy is directly related to energy intake!

Bone mineral density indicates how strong the bones are and how well they are hardening and developing, specifically in adolescents. Peak bone-mineral density is acquired by around age 19 for females and around age 20 for males. Low energy availability disrupts this process and, not surprisingly, increases the risk for stress fractures and early onset osteoporosis. In the case of 1) disordered eating or an eating disorder for at least 6 months and/or 2) recurring stress fractures, it is recommended that you get a bone density scan to assess bone health. It's important to be proactive and preventive, since bone fractures occurring prior to menopause are strong indicators of bone fractures after menopause. For athletes, low bone-mineral density may present an additional threat by restricting participation and performance in their sport. Furthermore, low bone-mineral density may not be fully reversible, despite efforts to increase energy intake, restore weight, and/or increase calcium and vitamin D intake.

This is especially true for those experiencing longer periods of low energy availability.

These changes in menstrual function and bone mineral density occur as a result of hormonal changes associated with low energy availability. As mentioned earlier, luteinizing hormone (LH) is responsible for ovulation. However, inadequate energy intake interferes with the LH release from the pituitary gland, and ovulation may be prevented. Low estrogen levels result from a lack of ovarian stimulation and can also be related to low body fat. This decline in estrogen levels contribute to low bone-mineral density in addition to a decline in other bone formation markers. This is exacerbated by a limited supply of nutrients that support bone formation (such as protein, calcium, and vitamin D). Low estrogen also negatively impacts the ability of the arteries to relax and allow greater blood-flow. Because arteries are responsible for delivering oxygenated blood from the heart to the body, this disturbance means a decrease in oxygen delivery to the muscles. As you can imagine, this interferes with optimal physical performance and health, including an increased risk for cardiovascular disease.

As mentioned above, RED-S identifies more consequences of low energy availability beyond that of menstrual dysfunction and bone density issues to include: decreases in endurance performance and muscle strength, a decreased ability to respond to training, increased irritability and risk for depression, increased risk of injuries, impaired growth and development, impaired metabolism, impaired immunity, increased cardiovascular risks and gastrointestinal issues, hormonal issues, and decreased ability to concentrate. Energy deficiency compromises many systems of the body in females AND males. If you are athlete attempting to gain a competitive edge by being thinner and restricting calories, I hope you see how these efforts compromise your performance goals.

Regardless of the mechanism or consequence of low energy availability, treatment is the same: consume more energy. Supply the body with adequate fuel.

FOOD IS FUEL

Your body needs fuel to function optimally. It relies on it. Without adequate energy, you are compromising that function. You may be able to survive on low calories for a time, but at what cost? We investigated some of the consequences above. Now think about what you gain and achieve from food as your fuel. Think about what matters to you.

You can have energy throughout the day, not feeling sluggish and lethargic. You can be productive and efficient in your workday or upbeat and energetic for your family and friends. Thoughts about food may no longer disrupt your sleep pattern. The continual irritability will dissipate as you experience a greater sense of well-being. One of the most common comments I receive from families when their family member has sufficiently increased energy intake is "I feel like I have my son/daughter/spouse back." If you are in treatment for mental health, adequate energy supports brain function to promote valuable work with your therapist, as well.

For athletes, you can achieve peak performance through developing greater strength and endurance. With adequate fuel, the tissues of your body and the physiological mechanisms in place for sports performance are supported. Many athletes are focused on muscle building and growth, which only happens when fueled by more calories than those that are expended. Just as you can't build a wall without a construction team and materials, you can't build your body without the necessary energy and nutrients (such as protein). Endurance-athletes need fat and carbohydrate stores. These need to be developed through adequate fuel, as well as the necessary training to maintain performance for longer periods of competition. In an interview with sport and performance psychologist Dr. Sari Shepphird, Ph.D., Lynn Bjorklund (an elite, long-distance runner who set U.S. records in high school and in young adulthood) describes this benefit of recovery and nutrition: "As an athlete, you are finally free to enjoy your sport the way it was meant to be. You are able to listen to your body with honesty, rather than denial, and take care of it such that you truly can be the very best that you can be for all the right reasons."

Moreover, fueling the body means supporting hormone levels that control vital functions of the body, including those that relate to menstrual function, bone health and cardiovascular health. The hormones that control hunger and satiety cues can normalize, leading to a trusting relationship with your body. Instead of the number of calories driving your eating pattern, your eating can be in response to physiological cues.

**Food is fuel for your body,
your mind, and your spirit.**

HOW TO FOCUS ON FOOD AS ENERGY

- Stop tracking your calories, especially using an app to do so. If you need to increase your calories for weight restoration, sport, and/or medical reasons, work with a registered dietitian nutritionist (RDN).

- Stop reading EVERY food label for calorie information.

- When eating at a restaurant, don't look up the nutrition information prior to ordering so you can base your decision on a number. Even better, don't go to a restaurant where calorie information is posted.

- Allow yourself to choose a high calorically-dense food (meaning a food that provides a larger amount of energy in a small amount of food). Focus on the taste and experience of eating.

- Eat a pre-workout snack and a recovery meal or snack within 15-20 minutes after exercise (possibly during if you are engaged in an endurance sport). Practice fueling.

- Don't eat ONLY because you have been exercising; maintain a steady daily eating pattern.

- Don't get on the scale and weigh yourself compulsively, most especially after a meal.

RECIPES

OVERNIGHT OATMEAL

SERVES 2

INGREDIENTS

1 cup rolled oats

2 cups milk (or almond milk)

2 bananas, mashed

2 tablespoons almond or peanut butter

Dash of cinnamon

¼ cup walnuts (optional)

¼ cup raisins (optional)

INSTRUCTIONS

1. Distribute ½ cup oats and 1 cup milk each into 2 separate small bowls.

2. Add 1 mashed banana, 1 tbsp nut butter, dash of cinnamon, handful of walnuts, and handful of raisins to each bowl. Stir to combine well.

3. Cover bowls and place in refrigerator overnight. Enjoy cold or heat in microwave for 1 minute in the morning.

Contributed by Katie Nili

GO-GET-'EM GRANOLA
SERVES 8

INGREDIENTS

1 ½ cups oats

2 cups nuts/seeds (your choice of nuts and seeds)

3 tablespoons coconut oil

¼ cup maple syrup

2 tablespoons honey

1 teaspoon vanilla extract

½ teaspoon almond extract

     (Can be substituted with another ½ teaspoon vanilla extract)

¼ teaspoon sea salt + extra for sprinkling

¼ teaspoon cinnamon, or to taste

¼ teaspoon pumpkin pie spice, or to taste

Optional: ¼ cup unsweetened dried coconut flakes

Optional: ¼ cup mix-ins (dried cranberries, dark chocolate chunks, etc.)

INSTRUCTIONS

1. Preheat oven to 300ºF.In a large mixing bowl, combine oats and nuts/seeds. Set aside for later.

2. In a microwave-safe bowl, combine coconut oil, maple syrup, honey, vanilla extract, almond extract, and ¼ teaspoon salt. Microwave for 1 minute. Stir mixture until coconut oil is completely melted or microwave for additional time, as needed.

3. Pour liquid mixture into oat/nut mixture. Stir until evenly coated.

4. Spread contents onto a baking pan lined with parchment paper. Pack down with a spatula.

5. Sprinkle mixture with sea salt, cinnamon, and pumpkin pie spice.

6. Place in the oven and bake for 20 minutes. Rotate tray 180º and bake for an additional 15-20 minutes or until golden brown.

7. Remove pan from the oven and let completely cool.

8. Break into chunks and add mix-ins as desired.

9. Serve over yogurt, as cereal, or on its own. It's delicious any way you serve it!

10. Store remaining granola in an airtight container. (If there's any left after the first taste!)

NOTES
I typically double the recipe. It fills a 13" x 9" pan.

Roast to your liking. I prefer my granola on the toasty side, so I typically bake it for a total of 40-45 minutes or until right before it begins to burn.

Experiment with different ingredients, spices, or extracts to find your perfect recipe. Use seasonal ingredients for optimal results or go wild and throw in some dried pineapple in the middle of December. It's granola. Just like life and body composition, you don't have to conform to society's standards to be fantastic!

Contributed by Sydney Fox
"For enjoying, energizing, and empowering yourself at any time of the day!"

QUINOA SALAD WITH DRIED CRANBERRIES AND FETA

SERVES 6

INGREDIENTS

4 cups of quinoa (pronounced as *kinwa*), cooked and cooled

2 green onions, finely sliced

½ large cucumber, sliced and quartered

¼ cup walnuts, toasted

¼ cup dried cranberries

1/3 cup Feta cheese, crumbled

1 cup baby spinach, roughly chopped

2 tablespoons extra virgin olive oil

2 tablespoons balsamic vinegar

1 tablespoon lemon juice

Salt and pepper to taste

Fresh basil (optional)

INSTRUCTIONS

1. Combine the cooked and cooled quinoa in a large bowl with onions, cucumber, walnuts, dried cranberries, feta cheese and spinach.

2. In a separate small bowl, combine the olive oil, balsamic vinegar, and lemon juice; mix well.

3. Pour the dressing over the salad and toss well. Season with salt and pepper, as desired.

4. Refrigerate for at least an hour.

5. Garnish with torn basil before serving.

Contributed by E.B.
Recipe from Nutrition by Bru and JamieGeller.com

GREEK YOGURT PARFAIT

SERVES 1

INGREDIENTS

1 cup Greek yogurt

1 cup fruit of choice

½ cup Go-Get-'Em Granola (or granola of choice)

Honey, to taste

INSTRUCTIONS

1. Add ½ cup Greek yogurt to a bowl, cup or other container.

2. Top with ½ cup fruit.

3. Top with ¼ cup granola.

4. Repeat steps 1-3, then drizzle with honey.

5. Dig in and enjoy!

Contributed by Sydney Fox

PUMPKIN PIE OATMEAL

SERVES 4

INGREDIENTS

1 cup old-fashioned roll oats

1 ¾ cups almond milk

¼ cup pumpkin puree

½ teaspoon vanilla extract

½ teaspoon ground cinnamon

¼ teaspoon ground nutmeg

½ cup chopped pecans

¼ cup maple syrup

INSTRUCTIONS

1. Combine oats and milk in a small saucepan over medium heat.

2. Bring to a boil; reduce heat and simmer, stirring occasionally until desired consistency is reached, about 3-5 minutes. Stir in pumpkin, vanilla extract, cinnamon and nutmeg until heated through, about 1 minute.

3. Serve immediately, garnished with pecans and maple syrup.

Contributed by Lauren Bohner
Recipe from damndelicious.net by Chungah Rhee

2

THE BENEFITS OF CONSUMING CARBS

When I ask friends and clients about dietary behaviors, one of the first comments I hear is, "I'm watching my carbs." Just as the word "calories" has become demonized, "carbs" has also become vilified. It's a nutrition topic that elicits fear and confusion for many. Numerous popular and fad diets (Ketogenic, Paleo, Atkins) promote limiting carbohydrates, which greater affirms one's decision to restrict carbohydrates for health and weight-related goals.

Carbohydrates, however, should be a part of a HEALTHY diet, one that promotes adequate energy, sports performance, digestive health, brain function, longevity, and quality of life. While the term "carbohydrates" is often associated with just bread and pasta, carbs are also found in beans, vegetables, starchy vegetables (such as sweet potatoes), fruit, dairy products, and grains (such as rice). Restricting carbohydrates means restricting rich sources of nutrition.

A MAJOR SOURCE OF ENERGY

The major role of carbohydrates in the body is to provide energy; it's the greatest source of fuel for your cells. This is especially evident when looking at the chemical process of metabolism in the body. The end products of metabolism are ATP (adenosine triphosphate), water, and carbon dioxide. ATP is known as the major energy compound in the body, fueling processes that keep you functioning. While carbohydrates, protein, and fat are all energy-yielding nutrients (meaning they can be metabolized to provide ATP), take a look at the figure below to see the major driver of ATP.

What's important to note is the compound at the top of the chain, glucose, which moves the energy cycle forward. Where does glucose come from? Carbohydrates.

Complex carbohydrates are built from chains of glucose molecules, including starches from grains and vegetables. On the other hand, *simple* carbohydrates are single, or at most two glucose molecules linked together. Simple carbohydrates include sugar found in fruits, dairy products, some vegetables, and table sugar. When not enough carbohydrate is available from these sources, your body will break down protein (muscle) in order to provide the necessary glucose for energy needs. This becomes important for maintaining a healthy blood glucose (or blood sugar) level, since a severe drop in blood glucose can be fatal. Therefore, one of the roles of consuming adequate carbohydrates is to spare using protein for energy needs. It is beneficial to eat enough carbohydrates to minimize the reliance on protein to provide glucose; protein must be preserved for other essential roles that can only be fulfilled by protein.

The brain relies on glucose for energy. In fact, it uses approximately 20% of the energy yielded by glucose in the body. Functions of the brain, such as memory, learning, focus, and concentration are linked to brain glucose levels. Limited glucose inhibits the production of neurotransmitters, the chemicals that carry messages in the brain. A key reason glucose is the preferred energy source for the brain is due to the presence of what's known as the *blood brain barrier*. The junctions between the cells of the blood-brain barrier are extremely tight. That leaves little room for certain compounds to pass from the blood to the brain. However, glucose can cross that barrier. Next time you consume carbohydrates, visualize that energy feeding your brain and your mind.

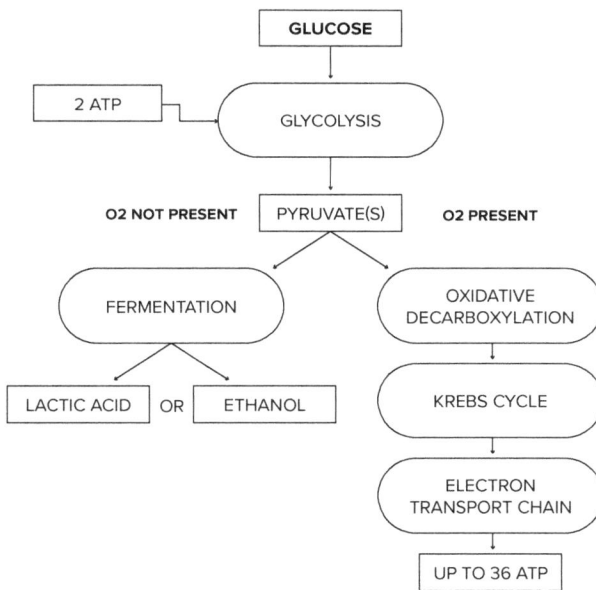

Flow of the Energy Chain

CARBS FOR EXERCISE

Carbohydrates are also fuel for exercise, which is especially important for endurance exercise and high-intensity workouts for the muscles. Carbohydrate is stored in the form of glycogen in both the liver and the muscles. The muscles hold approximately 1200-1600 calories worth of carbohydrates (energy!). These stores can be broken down rapidly for a quick source of energy when needed, such as during a sprint, yet can be a limiting factor for endurance athletes when not enough is available. Endurance performance is strengthened by having larger glycogen stores and the ability to preserve those stores by providing adequate carbohydrate intake. If you've ever heard the term "hitting the wall," this is a condition of sudden fatigue during endurance exercise when muscle and liver glycogen stores have been depleted.

Consumption of carbohydrates is recommended before, during, and after exercise sessions. Before an exercise session, carbohydrates help to top off stores of glycogen in the muscles. During exercise, they aid in maintenance of blood glucose levels, sparing your carbohydrate stores and increasing time until exhaustion. Carbohydrate consumption after exercise has several benefits, including enhanced rehydration when consumed with liquids, increasing the rate of muscle glycogen storage, and improving muscle recovery and rebuilding.

NUTRITIONAL BENEFITS OF HIGH CARBOHYDRATE FOODS

While carbs carry a negative label in our society, and especially in the weight loss industry, they have significant nutritional benefits. My clients are often surprised by the amount of nutrients various high-carbohydrate foods and beverages contain. In this book, it would be challenging to discuss all sources of carbohydrates and every nutrient provided in every food and beverage, so I'll just highlight some of them. As I discuss the nutritional value of foods, I'll refer to the Percent Daily Values (DV). These percentages are used to present the nutrients in one serving of a food or beverage item and are based on a 2000 calorie diet. For example, if a food label lists 30% DV for iron, it means that one serving of that food item provides 30% of your daily need for iron.

GRAINS

There are many different grains, each with its own distinct nutrient profile. Wheat is certainly one of the most vilified grains, partly due to its abundance in food products (such as bread, pasta, and snack foods) and partly due to the popularity of anti-wheat books such as, "Wheat Belly," and "Grain Brain." However, whole-grain wheat is a good source of protein, iron, magnesium, phosphorus, zinc, and vitamins B1 (thiamin) and B3 (niacin). And, it's an excellent source of fiber, an important contributor to gut health, as will be discussed later.

Whole grains also provide antioxidants to the body, which contribute to a decrease in inflammation and the risk of chronic diseases associated with inflammation. The United States Department of Agriculture (USDA) recommends that at least half of your grains should be whole grains.

Then there are the refined grains, whole grains that have been processed by removing the bran and germ components of the grain. The bran is rich in fiber and the germ is a rich source of nutrients, especially healthy fats. Most of these refined grains are enriched, meaning that some nutrients lost during processing are added back, leading to grains that are excellent sources of B vitamins (such as

B1, B2, and B3), iron, and folate. While a healthy diet pattern shouldn't be based on refined grains alone, there is room for them in a healthy diet—in moderation.

Other grains include barley, bulgur, rice, oats, and quinoa. Barley is rich in a soluble fiber called *beta glucan*, which helps lower cholesterol levels. Bulgur is a wheat-based grain that is especially high in fiber, providing approximately 8 grams per cup (the daily recommendation for fiber is 21-38 grams, depending on age and gender). Both brown and wild rice are whole grains. As is true with refined wheat, white rice is often enriched to provide greater nutritional value. Oats, commonly consumed in the form of oatmeal, are, as with barley, a rich source of beta glucan. As mentioned above, this type of soluble fiber is effective for lowering cholesterol. More recently, an antioxidant called *avenanthramides* has been recognized in oats, which may help protect your blood vessels from damage and inflammation that contribute to heart disease.

Quinoa is unique due to its protein content. This grain contains all nine essential amino acids (the building blocks of protein), making it a high-quality source of protein, similar to animal-based protein (meat, chicken, eggs, etc.). Essential amino acids are those that your body can't make on its own. Therefore, they must be provided in your diet. Quinoa is also classified as an ancient grain, a class of grains gaining popularity over the past few years. While there is no official definition of ancient grains, the Whole Grains Council defines ancient grains loosely as "grains that are largely unchanged over the last several hundred years." Other ancient grains include farro, teff, millet, spelt, kamut, sorghum, and amaranth, among others. Farro is especially high in zinc, B vitamins, and fiber, and has as nuttier flavor than many other grains. One cup of cooked amaranth provides 29% DV for iron, 9 grams of protein, and 5 grams of fiber. The chart below provides more information on the nutrient content of various grains. While it may seem compelling to limit yourself to eating only ancient grains, it's important to remember that each grain has a different nutrient profile and different nutritional strengths. Additionally, amaranth, buckwheat, millet, quinoa, wild rice, sorghum, teff, and oats (not contaminated with wheat during processing) are all gluten-free grains. The increasing availability of these grains has been incredibly valuable for those with celiac disease, those with an autoimmune response to gluten. However, the growth of the gluten-free food industry has also been perpetuated by the gluten-free diet craze. Some of my clients have used misinformation about gluten to restrict their food choices unnecessarily. Those that benefit from gluten-free eating include those with celiac disease, those that have an allergic response to wheat, or have non-celiac gluten sensitivity (NCGS) or what's more commonly referred to as gluten intolerance. Interestingly, current research seems to point to an intolerance to other fermentable carbohydrates versus the gluten in grain products (for those that complain of GI symptoms like cramping, bloating, diarrhea, and stomach pain). Avoiding gluten for the purpose of "eating healthier" is simply a way to engage in restricting behavior and participate in the dieting culture.

Grains (chart 1 columns): amaranth, buckwheat, cornmeal, millet, oats, quinoa, brown rice, sorghum, teff, wild rice

Nutrients (rows):
protein
fiber
iron
magnesium
phosphorus
zinc
copper
manganese
selenium
thiamin (B1)
riboflavin (B2)
niacin (B3)
pyridoxine (B6)
folic acid (B9)

Grains (chart 2 columns): bulgur, Kamut®, spelt, wheat, durum, wheat, red, wheat, white, barley, rye, triticale

Nutrients (rows):
protein
fiber
iron
magnesium
phosphorus
zinc
copper
manganese
selenium (na)
thiamin (B1)
riboflavin (B2)
niacin (B3)
pyridoxine (B6)
folic acid (B9)

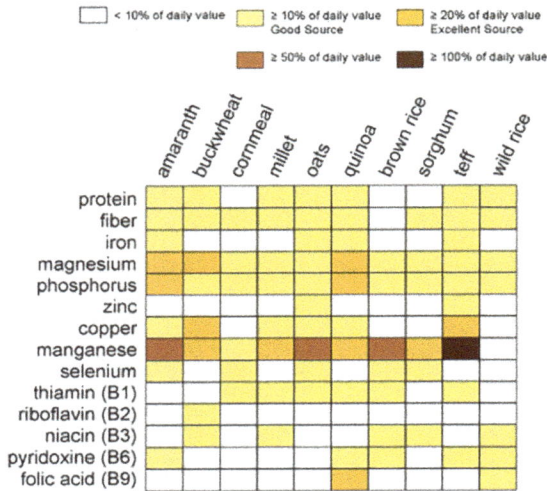

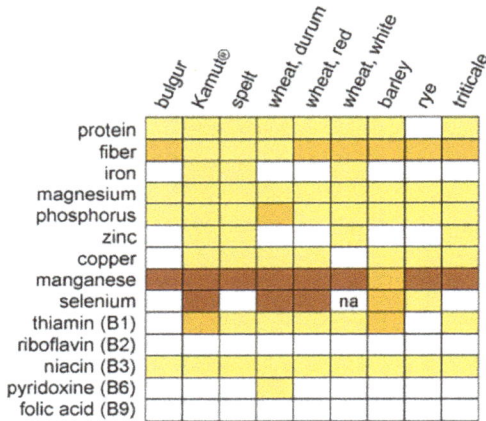

Nutrients Provided by Different Grains
(based on 45 grams or just under 1 cup serving)
Courtesy of the Oldways Whole Grains Council and www.wholegrainscouncil.org

STARCHY VEGETABLES

Starchy vegetables are those that are higher in carbohydrate content.

Unfortunately, they, too, have an unsupported bad reputation. These vegetables, as with non-starchy vegetables, have significant nutritional value. Potatoes provide a significant source of dietary fiber (4 grams in a medium baked potato), vitamin C (28% DV), potassium (26% DV; even more than a banana!), plus other nutrients like iron, magnesium, and B vitamins. Sweet potatoes are extremely high in vitamin A, in the form of beta carotene.

Corn, another starchy vegetable, is a significant source of dietary fiber, vitamin C, and the B vitamins folate and thiamin. It also contains the phytochemicals lutein and zeaxanthin. According to the American Optometric Association, these phytochemicals have been shown to be beneficial for eye health, decreasing the risk for age-related macular degeneration and cataracts. It is an antioxidant-rich vegetable, playing a role in sequestering free radicals that cause damage in your body. Free radicals are unstable atoms that act like scavengers—searching for hydrogen atoms. They contribute to aging and illness. Antioxidants help stabilize these free radicals by providing them with the necessary hydrogen, rendering the free radicals harmless.

FRUITS AND VEGETABLES

Thankfully, fruits and vegetables are typically less controversial. They're a valuable addition to your diet to meet many of your nutrient requirements. You don't need to avoid any specific ones, unless indicated by a specific medical issue, such as a food allergy, intolerance, or kidney disease. For example, I often hear faulty concerns from clients about bananas and carrots. They've been exposed to articles and peer opinions expressing concern over sugar content and their associated health risks.

A medium-sized banana provides 12% DV for potassium, 17% DV for vitamin

C, and 22% DV for vitamin B6. Bananas are a good source of dietary fiber and prebiotics, which feed the healthy bacteria in your gut, promoting digestive health. Likewise, one cup of carrots provides over 3 grams of dietary fiber, is an excellent source of vitamin K, provides 12% DV for potassium, and provides 428% DV of vitamin A as beta carotene.

It is well established that diets high in fruits and vegetables are associated with reduced chronic disease risk. You don't need to place restrictions on what to avoid in those food groups (again, unless warranted by specific medical issues). A large body of research supports the health benefits of plant-based diets that emphasize a **wide variety** of daily fruits and vegetables. Be purposeful about planning different fruits and vegetables into your meal plans and recipes.

OVERALL BENEFITS OF CARBOHYDRATES

Evidence of the nutritional benefits of carbohydrates is abundant. Studies support carbohydrates as a component of a healthy diet that may decrease risk of disease and death. A review of evidence from several studies, conducted in 2018, concluded that a moderate intake of carbohydrates (defined as 50-55% of energy intake) minimized risk of death. Less than 40% of energy from carbohydrates was associated with greater mortality risk. Authors concluded this observation was likely due to diets high in nutrient-rich food sources, such as whole grains and vegetables.

Another 2018 study investigated the impact of a healthy diet on brain size. Larger brain volume is associated with better cognitive function and better memory, whereas degeneration of areas of the brain (in size and functionality) is associated with neurological diseases like dementia. Authors of this study reported that a diet that is high in fruits, vegetables, whole grains, and dairy, along with nuts and fish, was associated with greater brain volume. A diet that included high-carbohydrate food sources (fruits, vegetables, whole grains, and dairy) was associated with better brain health. Additionally, the Iowa Women's Study found that women who consumed the greatest amount of whole grains had a greater than 35% reduction in risk of death associated with inflammatory diseases. Underlying inflammatory diseases contribute to conditions like diabetes, heart disease, chronic obstructive pulmonary disorder (COPD), asthma, emphysema, and Alzheimer's. There are numerous studies that continue to support inclusion of carbohydrates in a healthy diet.

FEEDING THE GUT

A final and important benefit of consuming adequate carbohydrates is how they contribute to digestive health. High carbohydrate foods, especially whole grains, fruits, vegetables, and legumes (such as beans and lentils) are significant sources of dietary fiber. Fiber can't be digested or absorbed by your body, because you don't have enzymes to break them down. And yet, they are beneficial for digestive health.

Insoluble fiber adds bulk and it draws water into your digestive system to promote bowel movements. Additionally, it speeds up the movement of your food through your large intestine, decreasing the transit time. Therefore, a diet that is high in insoluble fiber can be effective for preventing constipation. The muscles of your intestine have to work to move things along. It's weight-lifting for the intestinal muscles as we discussed earlier.

Soluble fiber dissolves in water, forming a gel-like substance. Because of this consistency, it traps cholesterol, helping to decrease blood cholesterol levels over time and lowering risk for heart disease. Soluble fiber may also help to stabilize blood sugar levels, which is important for those with diabetes or metabolic syndrome. Some soluble fibers are fermented by the bacteria living in your large intestine. These function as prebiotics—compounds that *feed* the bacteria in your gut. (This is different from probiotics—foods or supplements that *contain* live bacteria and yeast). Consumption of prebiotics has many researched benefits, and studies continue to identify specific actions of various prebiotics. These benefits include a decrease in inflammation associated with inflammatory bowel disease (IBD) and reduction of diarrhea while undergoing treatment for infection and taking an antibiotic. Additionally, the gut bacteria release fatty acids through the process of fermentation of these fibers. This action stimulates the release of hormones that promote satiety (feeling satisfied with your food and reducing hunger cues) and assist with blood sugar control. Research has reported that, on the other hand, lower levels of these fatty acids are associated with Type II diabetes and heart disease. Furthermore, if your body is underfed, this changes the composition of your gut microbiome. This has been correlated with an increased risk for anxiety and depression as evidence of the gut-brain axis (the communication between the nervous and digestive systems).

Another fiber-like substance is called *resistant starch*. Resistant starch opposes the work of your digestive enzymes, allowing that starch to enter the large intestine unchanged. This is beneficial in the same ways that soluble fiber is, including the production of fatty acids through the process of fermentation by intestinal bacteria. Resistant starch is found in plant cell walls and significant sources of resistant starch include both potatoes and pasta that have been cooked and then cooled.

Finally, a more diverse diet has been shown to lead to more diverse bacteria, which is beneficial for signaling the various systems of the body, including your immune system, gastrointestinal system, nervous system and endocrine system (in charge of your hormones). Different carbohydrates and nutrients promote a variety of healthy bacteria, meaning a variety in your food choices is a good thing!

With this understanding of carbs, you can welcome back the smell of baking bread.

HOW TO START CONSUMING CARBS

- Start your day with a carbohydrate-rich breakfast such as whole grain muffins, waffles, pancakes or cereal. All of these can be combined with nutritious fat sources like nuts and nut butters. You'll be well fueled and energized for the day ahead.

- If you have a significant fear about eating grains, start by adding them to a vegetable-based meal. A good example is sprinkling a salad with quinoa or even rice.

- Consume a starch or grain as a small portion of your meal, such as a side of pasta or rice. It can be overwhelming to have an entire plate of pasta in front of you if you haven't eaten pasta in a long time.

- Mix vegetables with your grains, such as broccoli mixed into a rice dish.

Again, this may help reduce uneasy feelings around the presence of grains. Creating a delicious stir fry is a great way to approach this!

- Challenge yourself by substituting a vegetable-based "rice," crust or "pasta" with the grain-based version. For example, substitute a cauliflower pizza crust with a traditional, fresh pizza dough.

- Create a baked potato loaded with vegetables and protein, such as cheese, broccoli, salsa, and chicken.

- Create a bowl with quinoa or rice as the base. Add vegetables, olive oil, and protein to create a simple meal. Quinoa has a reputation as a health food, making it easier for some people to consume.

- Create a bell-pepper dinner, stuffed with a mixture that includes rice and protein. Searching for a new recipe can be helpful with this.

- Choose a high carbohydrate snack, such as a piece of fruit, a smoothie, popcorn, or whole grain crackers. You can also create your own trail mix with nuts, dried fruit, and whole grain cereal.

RECIPES

GNOCCHI WITH SAUSAGE AND SPINACH
SERVES 2

INGREDIENTS

8 ounces store-bought potato gnocchi

2 tablespoons olive oil

4 ounces raw Italian sausage (casings removed) or bacon

Handful spinach (roughly chopped)

2 chopped garlic cloves

¼ cup unsalted butter

2 tablespoons shredded Pecorino-Romano cheese

1 teaspoon black pepper

INSTRUCTIONS

1. Cook gnocchi in a pot of boiling, salted water as instructed on the package. When complete, drain gnocchi, reserving 2 tbsp cooking water and set aside.

2. Heat olive oil in a skillet over medium-high heat. Add sausage (or bacon), and stir until sausage (or bacon) is cooked, about 4 minutes. Add spinach and cook until wilted, about 1 minute. Add garlic and cook until it is golden, about 1 minute.

3. Remove from heat, stir in butter and reserved gnocchi water. Add cooked gnocchi and toss until thoroughly mixed.

4. Stir in cheese and pepper.

Contributed by Katie Nili
Recipe adapted from Runner's World Magazine

LEMON BASIL PASTA

SERVES 4-6

INGREDIENTS

8 ounces linguine or other pasta

2 tablespoons melted margarine or butter

1 tablespoon fresh lemon juice

1 ½ teaspoon basil

¾ teaspoon garlic salt

¼ teaspoon black pepper

¼ cup grated Parmesan cheese

INSTRUCTIONS

1. Cook pasta according to package directions, omitting salt in cooking water.

2. Drain pasta and return to pan. In a small bowl combine butter, lemon juice, basil, garlic salt and pepper.

3. Toss with cooked pasta, chicken and shrimp can be added also.

4. Sprinkle cheese over pasta and serve immediately.

Contributed by E.B.
"This pasta is so very good. I've served it to people throughout the years and everyone loves it."

THE BEST MACARONI AND CHEESE EVER
SERVES 8

INGREDIENTS

1 (8-ounce) package (or 2 cups) elbow
    macaroni, cooked and drained

2 tablespoons butter

1 clove garlic, crushed

1 teaspoon onion powder

2 cups whole milk

1/4 cup all-purpose flour

6 cups sharp cheddar cheese

2 cups panko breadcrumbs

1/2 cup butter, melted

INSTRUCTIONS

1. Preheat oven to 400°F. In a large saucepan, melt the 2 tablespoons of butter, add the garlic and cook until the garlic is softened, about 2 minutes.

2. Add the onion powder, then whisk in the flour and milk, then cook until slightly thickened.

3. Add three cups of the cheddar cheese and stir until melted in the mixture.

4. Toss the cheese mixture with the cooked pasta, salt and pepper to taste. Stir the remaining grated cheese into the pasta. Spoon into a large baking dish.

5. In a small bowl, stir together the breadcrumbs and melted butter. (I always like to add a bunch of freshly ground pepper and a sprinkling of sea salt to this mixture.) Spread over the pasta.

6. Bake in a preheated oven for 20-25 minutes, or until the breadcrumbs are golden brown.

Contributed by Melody Kruse
"Macaroni and cheese has been one of my favorite foods since I was a kid. Learning to eat intuitively has taught me that it is okay to have foods I love and enjoy, and that all foods really are good foods. No food is off limits for me anymore. When I was in the depths of my eating disorder, there were so many rules I had to follow. Now I'm learning to listen to my body and give it what it wants and needs!"
Recipe from Babble.com by Brooke McClay

SIMPLE SPINACH LASAGNA
SERVES 12

INGREDIENTS

1 tablespoon extra virgin olive oil

2 (10 ounce) packages frozen
   chopped spinach

½ onion, chopped

½ teaspoon dried oregano

½ teaspoon dried basil

2 cloves garlic, crushed

1 (32 ounce) jar spaghetti sauce

1 ½ cups water

2 cups low fat cottage cheese

1 (8 ounce) package part skim
   mozzarella cheese, shredded

¼ cup grated Parmesan cheese

½ cup chopped fresh parsley

1 teaspoon salt

1/8 teaspoon black pepper

1 egg

8 ounces lasagna noodles

INSTRUCTIONS

1. Preheat oven to 350°F (175°C).

2. Pour oil into a large pot over medium heat. Sauté spinach, onion, oregano, basil and garlic in the olive oil.

3. Pour in spaghetti sauce and water; simmer 20 minutes.

4. In a large bowl mix cottage cheese, mozzarella cheese, Parmesan cheese, parsley, salt, pepper and egg.

5. Place a small amount of sauce in the bottom of a lasagna pan. Place 4 uncooked noodles on top of sauce and top with layer of sauce. Add 4 more noodles and layer with 1/2 of the sauce and 1/2 of the cheese mixture, add 4 more noodles and repeat until all is layered, finishing with sauce.

6. Cover with foil and bake in a preheated oven for 55 minutes. Remove foil and bake another 15 minutes. Let sit 10 minutes before serving.

Contributed by E.B.
"This is the basic lasagna recipe I use. When I'm in a hurry, I omit the garlic and onion and just use Italian, garlic, and onion seasonings. It's yummy."
Recipe adapted from allrecipes.com

BLUEBERRY STREUSEL-TOPPED MUFFINS

SERVES 12 MUFFINS

INGREDIENTS

1 ¾ cups all-purpose flour	¾ cup buttermilk
2 ¾ teaspoons baking powder	1/3 cup canola oil
¾ teaspoon table salt	1 cup fresh or frozen blueberries
½ cup sugar	1 tablespoon flour
2 teaspoons grated orange or lemon peel	1 tablespoon sugar
1 large egg	

STREUSEL-TOPPING:

¼ cup sugar	½ teaspoon cinnamon
2 ½ tablespoons flour	1 ½ tablespoons butter

INSTRUCTIONS

1. Preheat oven to 400°F. Line muffin tins with muffin papers.

2. Lightly spoon the 1 ¾ cups of flour into measuring cups, leveling with a knife. Place in large bowl and combine with the baking powder, salt, sugar, and citrus peel. Make a well in the center of the mixture.

3. In a small bowl, whisk together the egg, buttermilk, and oil. Pour into the well in the dry ingredients, stirring just until moistened.

4. In another small bowl, combine the 1 tablespoon of flour and 1 tablespoon of sugar. Toss the blueberries in this mixture until they are well-coated. Gently fold the blueberry mixture into the batter. Spoon the batter into lined muffin tins, filling 2/3 full.

5. To make the streusel topping, combine the 1/4 cup sugar, 2 1/2 tablespoons flour, and ½ teaspoon cinnamon. Cut in the butter with a pastry cutter or two butter knives until the mixture is crumbly. Sprinkle over the batter and bake for 18 minutes or until the tops are golden and a toothpick inserted into the center of one of the muffins comes out clean.

6. Remove from oven and allow to cool in the pan for 5 minutes. Then transfer to a cooling rack.

Contributed by E.B.
"The orange zest adds a yummy addition, very satisfying. So much better than the box."
Recipe from ourbestbites.com by Kate Jones

PUMPKIN BREAD
SERVES 1 LOAF

INGREDIENTS

1 heaping cup flour

1 cup sugar

¾ teaspoon baking soda

½ teaspoon salt

⅓ teaspoon cinnamon

¾ cup canned pumpkin puree

⅓ cup vegetable oil

2 tablespoons water

1 egg

⅔ cup peanut butter chips or pumpkin chips

⅓ cup nuts (optional)

⅓ cup raisins (optional)

INSTRUCTIONS

1. Heat oven to 350°F.

2. Grease and flour 1 loaf pan.

3. In a medium bowl, combine flour, sugar, baking soda, salt, and cinnamon; set aside.

4. In a large mixing bowl, blend pumpkin puree, oil, water, and eggs.

5. Gradually add dry ingredients until well blended.

6. Stir in chips, nuts, and raisins. Pour into pre-greased pan.

7. Bake at 350 degrees for 45-50 minutes or until a toothpick comes out clean.

8. Cool loaf in pan for 10 min; remove from pan and completely cool on rack.

Contributed by Katie Nili

GREEK YOGURT FETTUCCINE ALFREDO
SERVES APPROXIMATELY 4-6

INGREDIENTS

1 pound (16 ounces) pasta noodles of choice

1 cup plain Greek yogurt

1 ½ cups grated parmesan cheese

1 egg, beaten

1 teaspoon salt

¼ cup olive oil

1-2 teaspoons dried basil

3-5 cloves garlic, minced

Optional: protein source of choice

INSTRUCTIONS

1. Bring a large pot of water to boil (with a pinch of salt and a drizzle of olive oil). Add pasta noodles of your choice and cook until al dente.

2. In a medium mixing bowl, combine the yogurt, grated parmesan, egg, and salt.

3. Add oil to a small saucepan on low heat, add basil and garlic and cook until fragrant and sizzling (not burnt!).

4. Drain the pasta and return to the pot. Add the oil mixture into the pasta and stir to completely coat the pasta.

5. Mix in yogurt sauce (and protein if using) until combined. Now... dig in!

Contributed by Sydney Fox
Recipe from colleenquigley.org by Colleen Quigley, an Olympic steeplechaser and national champion

APPLESAUCE MUFFINS

SERVES 12

INGREDIENTS

2 cups flour

1 teaspoon baking soda

1 teaspoon cinnamon

1 teaspoon allspice

1 teaspoon salt

1 cup sugar

½ cup shortening (or butter)

2 eggs

1 cup applesauce

Optional:

1 cup raisins

½ cup chopped nuts

INSTRUCTIONS

1. Heat oven to 350°F.

2. Cream together sugar and shortening.

3. Add eggs and cream until light and fluffy.

4. Add applesauce and mix well.

5. In another bowl, sift or stir together all other dry ingredients. Add to the applesauce mixture; beat until just blended.

6. Stir in raisins and nuts, if desired.

7. Spoon into muffin cups (fill half full). Bake 20 minutes or until golden brown. Serve warm or cold.

Contributed by E.B.
Recipe from Cooking Something Up Cookbook

RED BEANS AND RICE

SERVES 8

INGREDIENTS

1 pound dry red kidney beans, rinsed and sorted

6 cups chicken broth

1/3–1/2 pound smoked sausage (Andouille sausage, if you can find it), quartered and cut into thin slices. You can also use a large, meaty ham bone.

1 onion, chopped

4–5 cloves garlic, minced

1 teaspoon Cajun or Creole seasoning (Tony Chachere's is the best; omit this if using Andouille sausage)

3/4 teaspoon cumin

3/4 teaspoon coriander

3/4 teaspoon oregano

1/8 teaspoon cinnamon (sounds weird, but DON'T leave it out!!!)

1/2 teaspoon smoked paprika or liquid smoke to taste

RICE:

4 cups water

1 tablespoon white vinegar

2 cups white rice

INSTRUCTIONS

1. Combine all ingredients in a crock pot and cook on high for 4-5 hours or on low all day. You can start on high until it starts to simmer and then switch it to low. If you're at a high elevation, the beans will need to cook longer and/or you need to soak them overnight before you start cooking them in the morning.

2. When beans are tender, mash about 85-90% of them against the side of the crock pot. Give them a taste and add any extra seasonings if you need to, particularly more Tony's or salt and pepper. Replace lid and set heat to "low."

3. In a medium saucepan, bring 4 cups water, 1 tablespoon white vinegar, and 2 cups white rice to a boil. Reduce heat to low, cover, and steam for 20 minutes.

4. Serve beans with rice.

Contributed by E.B.
Recipe from ourbestbites.com by Kate Jones

3

THE FLAVOR OF FATS

I recall as a teenager in the 1990s watching Susan Powter on television talking about food and weight. Susan was a motivational speaker, author of diet and nutrition books, and host of *The Susan Powter Show*. Her message was: "It's fat that makes you fat!" She boomed this message to many Americans who were seeking weight loss results. Even now, it's a concept many people still believe. However, science has shown this idea to be inaccurate, since fat, in and of itself, does not cause weight gain. As the American Heart Association says," Fat gets a bad rap, even though it is a nutrient that we need in our diet."

Fat can promote a healthy heart, a healthy weight, and a healthy appreciation for the taste of food. Fat carries flavor! For example, visualize a plain, dry piece of toast. Now add something like butter, avocado, a drizzle of olive oil, or an olive tapenade. The taste and appeal of that toast changes. Plus, you'll feel more satisfied by that food option and less likely to look for something else. Fat should not be feared; it should be appreciated for the unique benefits it provides in your food and in your body.

HOW FATS BENEFIT THE BODY

One of the first roles of fats is to promote absorption of fat-soluble vitamins, including vitamins A, D, E, and K. Vitamin A plays an important role in your vision, including your ability to adapt to dim light. It's essential for reproductive function, immune function, and cell growth (an essential role during pregnancy).

Many people are familiar with the role of vitamin D in bone health. It promotes the absorption of calcium in your body and helps protect bone from breaking down. Moreover, it plays a role in cell growth and other specialized functions for certain cells. Vitamin D is also currently being studied for its relationship with autoimmune diseases, such as multiple sclerosis and lupus, and for a possible supportive role in cancer prevention.

Vitamin E is known for its contribution to your immune system, acting as an antioxidant. Vitamin K, as with vitamin D, is essential for bone health, contributing to the building of the bone. It is also important for blood-clotting, decreasing risk for excessive blood loss.

Consumption of adequate fat promotes the absorption of these vitamins found in your food, moving them from your GI tract to the rest of your body. Fat-soluble vitamins travel with fat rather than water. (When you look at a bottle of oil and vinegar salad dressing, you can see how the fat separates from the vinegar or watery part. Fat-soluble vitamins stay in the oil layer, not the vinegar.)

Therefore, when fat is absorbed from the intestines, it will carry the fat-soluble vitamins with it. By adding full-fat salad dressing, oil, avocado, or nuts to a salad, you will absorb more nutrients from the foods in your salad that contain fat-soluble vitamins. You get more "bang for your buck."

Fats are also an essential energy source, which is extremely important for dedicated athletes and recreational exercisers. Fats are stored in muscles and in adipose tissue, as well as in the form of free fatty acids that travel in the blood. They are especially important during aerobic and endurance exercise as fats are slowly released for energy. Fats in food provide a concentrated source of energy, which is helpful in keeping the volume of meals and snacks smaller. This is especially desirable if someone has high energy needs, as is the case with some athletes, or if the ability to eat is inhibited. For example, after a period of starvation and/or malnutrition, when nutritional restoration is necessary, it would be extremely challenging to restore without adequate use of fats. The volume of food would simply be too large and likely intolerable without significant intake of nutritious fats.

In Chapter 1, I spoke about the importance of fueling the body. Adequate fat intake is a key piece of getting that fuel. While you may fear weight-gain associated with eating fat, this nutrient helps promote satiety by slowing the release of food from your stomach. Satiety means being full or gratified; feeling satisfied. Years ago, I had a client report that she couldn't stop eating and never felt satisfied. This resulted in having a lack of control at meals, moving from one food to another due to ongoing hunger cues. After investigating her food journals, it was apparent that she avoided fat in her meals. By intentionally adding fat at all meals, she was better able to manage and satisfy her hunger, her eating behaviors improved, the taste of her food was more enjoyable, and she was able to focus on things outside of her next snack or meal.

Fat provides insulation to your body, helping you to stay warm. I commonly ask clients if they get cold easily, and those who are underweight will usually respond, "yes". Indeed, this is why those who have experienced severe weight loss will often complain of *lanugo*—a soft, fine hair that will develop on the skin as a way for the body to provide insulation. It's the body's way of providing protection in the absence of adequate fat. Furthermore, fat provides a protective cushioning layer around your vital organs. Although the health consequences of *excessive* levels of fat is widely agreed upon by health experts, especially as it relates to heart disease, this protective layer is important. It allows for shock absorption if you fall, decreasing your risk of injury. Additionally, you have a protective, fatty tissue called the *omentum*, which helps stabilize organs in their place, provides immunity, and promotes healing.

Finally, while adipose tissue is often recognized for its unlimited capacity for energy storage in the form of fat, it is also responsible for releasing hormones. Hormones are chemical substances that promote specific actions in the body, targeting different cells and tissues. Scientists now view adipose tissue as a major endocrine (hormone-producing) organ, like the pancreas. Adipose tissue releases several hormones, including *leptin* and *adiponectin*. Leptin is known to decrease hunger and helps to regulate the energy balance of the body, playing an important role in body-weight. Adiponectin plays a role in regulation of blood sugars and your cells' response to insulin (another hormone). Adipose tissue is also involved in your immunity, as well as the functioning of the reproductive system, based on the various hormones it releases or regulates.

Fat is essential to body function. It's not simply something that affects your waistline, as many people fear. Furthermore, fat, in the form of essential fatty acids, has a pivotal role in brain health and development. Your brain is approximately 60% fat; therefore, fat intake can significantly affect its functioning.

ESSENTIAL FATTY ACIDS

Essential fatty acids are those the body can't make on its own; they must be eaten. They include omega-3 fatty acids, such as *α-linolenic acid*, and omega-6 fatty acids, such as *α-linoleic acid*. (I know, the names are very similar!) Sources of omega-3 fatty acids include fish oil, ground flaxseed, walnuts, chia seeds, and canola oil. Sources of omega-6 fatty acids include safflower oil, sunflower seeds, pine nuts, and corn oil.

In the brain and throughout the body, these essential fatty acids are incorporated into cell membranes. They play a role in allowing molecules to pass into and out of the cell, protecting the cell and cell function. High levels of the omega-3 fatty acid DHA (*docosahexaenoic acid*) are found in the brain, leading to the idea that DHA is important in the function and development of that organ. Simply walk down the baby section at a grocery store and you'll note the multitudes of formulas with added DHA to promote healthy brain development.

While the use of this supplementation hasn't been conclusively backed by research, most experts recommend a daily intake of at least 200 mg of DHA during pregnancy, because the mother's intake determines the nutrient level in the baby. DHA also plays a role in the brain's communication pathways and system of neurotransmitters. Neurotransmitters are the chemical messengers of the nervous system. The importance of adequate levels is especially evidenced in the elderly—as omega-3 levels decline, memory and brain function also decline. Overall, the brain relies on adequate fat levels to communicate effectively from cell to cell.

Your vision is also dependent on DHA, since it is also found in the retina of the eye. The retina converts light into a signal that is sent to the brain, and the brain translates the signal into a picture of what you see.

Furthermore, essential fatty acids are important to your immune response and ability to decrease inflammation. There are different mechanisms by which these fatty acids accomplish that. Because of this anti-inflammatory role, omega-3 fatty acids are researched for possible benefits in disease management, such as rheumatoid arthritis and inflammatory bowel diseases.

Finally, it's important to note the relationship between essential fatty acids and heart health; likely the most talked about benefit of essential fatty acids through the media. The American Heart Association recommends consuming at least two servings (3.5 ounces each) of fatty fish each week. Fatty fish include salmon, tuna (especially albacore, although higher in mercury), sardines, trout, herring, and mackerel. These fish are significant sources of two types of omega-3 fatty acids, DHA and EPA (*eicosapentaenoic acid*). This recommendation is based on evidence indicating a reduced risk of death from coronary heart disease (due to an arrhythmia) and sudden cardiac death.

Additionally, studies show that an increased intake of DHA and EPA significantly reduces triglyceride levels in the blood. Triglycerides are essentially a type of fat, and high levels are considered an independent risk factor for heart disease. Therefore, those with high triglyceride levels may be candidates for fish oil supplementation. While much of the conversation on essential fatty acids and heart health is focused on omega-3 fatty acids, omega-6 fatty acids are associated with a reduction in blood cholesterol levels, as well. A 2012 meta-analysis concluded that an increase in omega-6 fatty acids leads to a reduction of coronary heart disease by 10%. Most American diets are more predominant in omega-6 fatty acids, therefore, focusing on omega-3 fatty acid intake is a more common dietary focus.

POLYUNSATURATED AND MONOUNSATURATED FATTY ACIDS

Omega-3 and omega-6 fatty acids are types of polyunsaturated fatty acids. Other sources high in polyunsaturated fatty acids are sunflower seeds, soybean oil, sesame seeds, and other vegetable oils. Monounsaturated fatty acids are found in avocados, olives and olive oil, nuts (such as peanuts, hazelnuts, almonds, pecans), nut butters, peanut oil, safflower oil, canola oil, and seeds.

Choosing these healthful fat sources can help to lower your total cholesterol and low-density lipoprotein cholesterol (LDL cholesterol), reducing your risk for heart disease. The Mediterranean-style diet emerged from the observation of lower heart disease rates among the people of Greece and other Mediterranean regions in the 1960s. Although they enjoy a high-fat diet, they consume higher levels of olive oil, which is high in monounsaturated fatty acids. Endorsements for following the Mediterranean-style diet as a way to improve health and decrease disease risk are abundant. It is recommended as a healthful diet approach by the American Heart Association, the Dietary Guidelines for Americans, and the World Health Organization. Additionally, olive oil is rich in antioxidants and there's a body of research indicating olive oil may help decrease inflammation, promote brain function, and reduce risk for Type II diabetes, especially as a part of the Mediterranean-style diet.

Bottom line: Fat is vital to a healthy life. Be intentional about cooking with olive oil, dipping vegetables into hummus, adding nuts to your cereal and salads, adding avocado to your sandwiches, and spreading nut butters on your morning toast. Restricting fat is not a healthful eating strategy.

CULINARY USE OF FATS

It is often suggested that the secret to French cooking is wrapped up in one word—butter. If you've ever watched Julia Child in action, you'll know what I mean. Butter and other fats provide flavor and palatability to foods, something you don't get from pure carbohydrates or protein. Fat is important if you are looking for pleasure in the eating experience.

Fat contributes a specific mouthfeel to foods and beverages, a richness that enhances flavor. For example, consider non-fat milk versus cream. Cream has a softer mouthfeel and richness, making it extremely palatable.

Furthermore, there are different chemical structures that contribute to flavor. Benzaldehyde is found in almonds, vanillin is responsible for the flavor of vanilla, and cinnamaldehyde contributes to the odor and flavor of cinnamon.

Fat contributes to the final texture of baked goods. As any baker will tell you, the creaming of fat with sugar produces a soft and fluffy baked item. Using butter creates a flaky pastry or biscuit and fat promotes tenderness in a product, making foods easier to cut and chew. During the baking process, fat interferes with the binding of protein strands (commonly gluten) in flour-based products, contributing to the product's tenderness.

Fat marbling in the muscle tissue of meat helps maintain moisture and tenderness. In salad dressings, fat acts as an emulsifier to produce an even consistency. As mentioned earlier, when you look at a bottle of salad dressing, you'll often see a separation between the oil and vinegar, with the oil floating at the top. However, when you shake that bottle, the particles evenly disperse, yielding an even consistency throughout the dressing, making it an emulsion. Mustard is often added to salad dressing as the emulsifying ingredient to keep the oil and vinegar from separating.

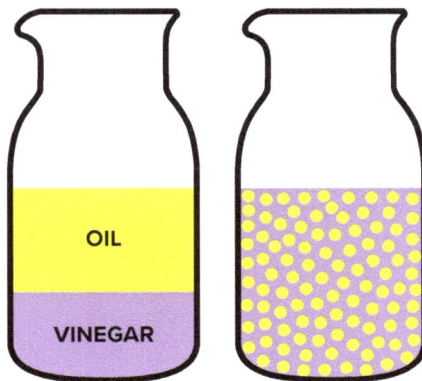

Example of an emulsion in a salad dressing

Finally, oil acts to conduct heat in the process of cooking. Oils can heat from around 350 degrees to just above 500 degrees, with some oils containing higher smoke points than others (in other words, the temperature at which the fat will start to burn and smoke). This is why it's important to choose the right oil when you are cooking at high temperatures, including stir frying. During frying, oils help to slightly dehydrate the food and, with that moisture loss, you get a crispy texture and delicious flavor!

I recognize that some of you may fear fats BECAUSE you know fat adds flavor and taste to your foods. That palatability lends to eating at a rapid pace, especially during an overeating or a binge eating episode. Once you've recognized that eating high-fat foods isn't something wrong or bad, start by slowing down. Eat in the presence of others and pay attention to what you are eating. Stay present during the eating experience.

Fat does not make you fat.
It is essential for health and
for your eating pleasure.

HOW TO ENJOY THE FLAVOR OF FATS

- Add a couple of spoonsful of avocado to your next sandwich, taco, toast, or salad. Many of my clients have had an easier time adding avocado as a fat option versus other sources of fat.

- Brush your fish, poultry, or meat with oil before grilling or brush your bread with oil to create a grilled sandwich. This keeps the portion small and contributes to the crispy texture.

- Drizzle salad dressing or a combination of oil and vinegar over your salad and toss to combine.

- Blend peanut butter or almond butter into a smoothie. One of my favorites is a peanut butter and frozen banana smoothie made with milk.

- Use nuts and seeds to top yogurt, oatmeal, or even waffles or pancakes at breakfast. This adds to the texture of the meal.

- Add salmon and tuna to your weekly meal routine. Get creative with recipes like salmon tacos or tuna noodle casserole.

- Use a serving of nut butter as a delicious dip for apples or spread it onto a banana. Individual packages of nut butter are now available at grocery stores that make it easy and convenient.

- Drizzle oil into a pan and use it to sauté vegetables. A little goes a long way to add flavor, texture and nutritional value to your vegetables!

RECIPES

AVOCADO TOAST

SERVES 1

INGREDIENTS

1 slice of toasted bread

1/4 avocado

1 slice cheese

1 fried egg

¼ cup spinach

INSTRUCTIONS

1. Place the slice of toasted bread on a plate and spread with the avocado.

2. Top with spinach, cheese and a fried egg for a scrumptious and tasty meal that is a great way to supply your body with all the nutrients it needs!

Contributed by Melody Kruse

"Since learning to embrace recovery from my eating disorder, I am learning to fall in love with food all over again. Avocado toast feels like a party in my mouth!"

BALSAMIC ROASTED BRUSSEL SPROUTS

SERVES 4

INGREDIENTS

1 pound Brussels sprouts

¼ cup olive oil

3 tablespoons balsamic vinegar (or to taste)

8-12 cloves garlic, minced or whole (to taste)

Sea salt

Ground black pepper

INSTRUCTIONS

1. Preheat oven to 425°F. Line a shallow baking pan with foil.

2. Trim off ends Brussels sprouts along with any loose outer leaves. Slice in half, lengthwise.

3. Place Brussels Sprouts, olive oil, vinegar, garlic, salt & pepper into a bowl and mix. Pour mixture out onto prepared baking pan.

4. Roast in oven for 20-25 minutes until tender, stirring occasionally.

Contributed by Sydney Fox

PEANUT CHICKEN PAD THAI

SERVES 3-4

INGREDIENTS

1 (12 ounce) package rice noodles

2 tablespoons sesame oil

2 cloves chopped garlic

1 cup shredded carrots

1 cup thinly sliced red cabbage

1 large red bell pepper, thinly sliced

2 large chicken breasts, cooked and
    shredded

Peanut sauce:

½ cup peanut butter

⅓ cup honey

⅓ cup soy sauce

2 tablespoons sesame oil

2 tablespoons rice vinegar

2 teaspoons fresh ginger

Optional Garnish:

Sesame seeds

Chopped cilantro

Chopped peanuts

Green onions

INSTRUCTIONS

1. Combine all ingredients for the peanut sauce in a small saucepan over low heat. Whisk until everything is melted and combined. Remove from heat and set aside.

2. Cook noodles according to package instructions and set aside.

3. Heat 2 tablespoons sesame oil and garlic in a skillet over medium heat. Add carrots, cabbage, and red bell pepper slices. Cook for about 5 minutes until the vegetables are slightly tender. Once tender, add the noodles and shredded chicken to the skillet. Remove from heat.

4. Pour peanut sauce over chicken and vegetables. Toss until combined. Top with sesame seeds, cilantro, peanuts, and green onion.

Contributed by Katie Nili
Recipe adapted from Pinterest

NUT BUTTER ENERGY BITES

SERVES APPROXIMATELY 10 BITES

INGREDIENTS

1 cup almond or peanut butter

6 dates

¼ cup cashews

½ teaspoon cinnamon

½ cup rolled oats

Coconut flakes (optional)

INSTRUCTIONS

1. Put all ingredients except coconut flakes in food processor and pulse until combined.

2. Roll mixture into the size and shape of golf balls. Roll in coconut flakes (optional).

Contributed by Katie Nili

PESTO SALMON

SERVES 4

INGREDIENTS

4 tablespoons basil pesto

2 tablespoons butter softened

1 garlic clove, zested

4 (7 ounce) salmon fillets

Salt & pepper to taste

1 teaspoon fresh lemon juice

INSTRUCTIONS

1. Preheat your oven to 400°F.

2. In a small bowl, combine the basil pesto, softened butter, and zested garlic using a fork. Set aside.

3. Line a baking sheet with foil and lay the salmon fillets on top. Generously season with salt and pepper and squeeze a little bit of lemon juice on top. (About 1/4 teaspoon per fillet)

4. Using a cookie scoop, place two scoops of the pesto mixture on each fillet.

5. Bake for 10 minutes.

Contributed by E.B.
Recipe adapted from simplyhomecooked.com by Dina Polyashov

4

THE POWER OF PROTEIN

In my experience, protein tends to be the "safe" and "good" nutrient as communicated by my clients and in social media. Commercials and food marketing campaigns are often focused on the protein content of products, evidenced by labels that state "high in protein," or "now with more protein." While people are concerned about getting enough protein in their diet, most Americans consume plenty of protein to meet their needs. This being said, I encounter many clients who will limit animal-based protein sources as an easy way to diet or restrict calories. Choosing to be vegetarian or vegan becomes a way to manipulate the diet that sounds healthy but reflects fear instead of knowledge.

There are definitely benefits of plant-based diets, substantiated by research, and I'm not opposed to vegetarian diets. However, it's important to make those decisions with the understanding of how animal-based protein sources fit into a healthy eating pattern and provide essential nutrients. It's also important to work with a dietitian to establish dietary strategies to meet your nutrient needs. Once you have a clear understanding of how all foods fit into a healthy diet, you can avoid fear-based decisions as you construct your long-term eating plan.

OUR BUILDING BLOCKS

Protein is the building material for most structures of the body. This includes collagen found in bones, muscles, skin and tendons. However, it also includes enzymes, hormones and antibodies. Protein turnover happens around the clock in the body, as cells are broken down, repaired and rebuilt, even in bones. Enzymes and hormones go through this process rapidly, being fully replaced within a few minutes to a few hours. This recycling process lends to the importance of protein intake—having adequate protein available for the individual needs of each body structure.

Proteins have other essential roles besides being used as structural material. They attract water, making them useful for maintaining fluid balance in the body. Refer to the figure below, which shows a malnourished child in a third-world country, where starvation is common. While she appears thin and frail, she has a distended belly, full of fluid that has leached into that space. This is because of protein malnutrition, a condition called *kwashiorkor*. Protein is also involved in the acid-base balance of the body, as protein acts as a buffer (to reduce acidity).

Additionally, proteins act as transporters throughout the body. For example, they help transport compounds through the fat-rich membrane that surrounds cells. Think of them as channels allowing passage in and out. They also carry fats throughout the blood, performing like taxis to get fats to their targeted tissues where they will be stored or used for fuel. Moreover, protein is used for energy, as it can enter the energy cycle shown in Chapter 1. In the absence of adequate carbohydrate in the diet, more protein will be used for energy, being converted to glucose. As discussed earlier, one of the benefits of consuming adequate carbohydrates is that is spares protein so it's available for its numerous other roles.

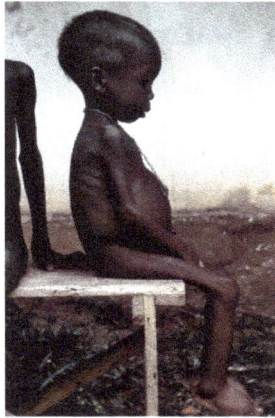

Starved Girl
Courtesy of Centers for Disease Control and Prevention

Proteins are made of chains of building blocks called amino acids. The sequence and structure of these amino acids determines the function of the protein. While there are many different biologically important amino acids, there are 20 that play vital roles in the body. Furthermore, 9 of those 20 are essential, meaning you must consume those amino acids from food sources, since your body can't create them on its own. If a food or beverage contains all 9 essential amino acids, it is labeled as a high-quality protein source. One of the nutritional strengths of animal-based protein sources is their amino acid content, as they provide all of the essential amino acids, while most plant sources do not. Plant sources of all nine essential amino acids are limited to soy, quinoa, and buckwheat.

One fascinating discovery in the body is amino acid "pools." Your body doesn't store protein as it does with carbohydrates and fats; however, amino acids need to be constantly available for the body to create the various protein-based structures and elements (such as enzymes and hormones). Therefore, your cells have these amino acid "pools", which yield readily available amino acids to be used during the construction process. Visualize a child's alphabet building blocks laid out on the floor, all mixed up (amino acid "pools"). When the child wants to string those blocks together to create a word (a protein structure), all of the letters contained in that word must be available for perfect completion. That line up of individual blocks now has meaning in the form of a word. Animal-based proteins help ensure that individual amino acids are available as needed by your body to build complete structures. Plant-based proteins contribute to the amino acid "pools," but a variety of sources must be eaten to ensure adequate amino acids are available, such as those from grains and legumes (think bread and peanut butter or rice and beans).

BENEFITS OF MEAT

As mentioned above, one of the main benefits of consuming meat is its protein content. When I ask clients what they know about meat, the common response is simply "it is high in protein." Beyond that nutritional strength, they are unable to identify additional nutrients. Whether you choose chicken, turkey, beef, or pork, they are all nutrient-rich sources.

Meat, especially red meat, is a strong source of heme iron. This form of iron is more available to the body for absorption and use, as opposed to iron found in plant-based sources. Examples include beef, chicken, turkey, pork and lamb. Additionally, the consumption of meat, fish, and poultry can enhance the availability of non-heme iron found in grains, beans, greens, and other plant-based sources. Iron is an integral part of many proteins and enzymes that help maintain good health; it is an essential component of the proteins that are involved in oxygen transport. It is also essential for the regulation of cell growth and differentiation (specialized cell function). A deficiency of iron limits oxygen delivery to cells, resulting in fatigue, poor work and exercise performance, and decreased immunity. Children with iron deficiency anemia have difficulty with growth and maturation, as well as cognitive function and learning. Because supplemental iron may lead to nausea and constipation, getting your iron from food sources is certainly desirable. Moderate amounts of meat can help you meet your iron requirements.

In addition to iron content, beef is a high source of vitamin B12, selenium, zinc, niacin, and vitamin B6. A 3-ounce portion of meat provides at least 20% DV of each of these nutrients. The B vitamins are important for energy production in your body; selenium acts as an antioxidant; and zinc is involved in your immune response. Furthermore, high concentrations of zinc are found in the brain and zinc status impacts both mental health and behavior. Zinc deficiency can perpetuate disordered eating and underfeeding contributes to zinc deficiency. It's a vicious cycle. Other consequences of zinc deficiency include alterations in taste and low appetite. There is strong evidence for including foods high in zinc content and yet the avoidance of meat is common among those dieting and engaging in disordered eating. Another nutrient found in beef is choline, which has drawn more attention in recent years, especially as a nutrient of importance during fetal development. Choline is essential during development of the brain and central nervous system and, therefore, plays a role in cognitive function and learning. Additionally, choline functions as a part of the neurotransmitter acetylcholine (a chemical messenger).

The nutritional content of pork is similar to beef but is also known to be an excellent source of the B vitamin, thiamin. Thiamin is critical for energy production and development of cells. Chicken breast is commonly acknowledged as a lean protein source. It is exceptionally high in niacin and vitamin B3, providing 57% DV in a 3-ounce serving. Chicken is an excellent source of vitamin B6 and selenium, and is also a good source of phosphorus— critical for the mineralization of bones and teeth and energy transfer in the body. Finally, turkey shares in the rich nutrient content of the other meats, providing vitamin B6, B12, niacin, choline, selenium, and zinc. While turkey is a significant source of the amino acid, tryptophan, it is not high enough to promote sleepiness, despite public myth.

Another intriguing note about meat and poultry is their leucine content, another amino acid. This is an important nutrition concept for athletes, since leucine is understood to be a trigger for muscle anabolism (the building of muscle protein) and recovery after exercise sessions. Experts recommend 20 grams of high-quality protein per meal, which would have adequate leucine to trigger this response. This can be provided in 2 ½ to 3 ounces of meat, a benefit of consuming meat for training and exercise performance.

Resistance to eating meat, and especially red meat, sometimes stems from health-related concerns. Therefore, it's important to address that here. The two most common concerns are 1) heart health or cardiovascular disease and 2) cancer. While many of my clients tend to think that nutrition habits are "all or nothing," research shows that red meat can be consumed in moderation. The American Institute for Cancer Research states: "The evidence that red meat (beef, pork, and lamb) is a cause of colorectal cancer is convincing. Studies show, however, that we can consume modest amounts—12 to 18 ounces (cooked) per week—without a measurable increase in colorectal cancer risk."

To put this in perspective, a 3-ounce portion of meat is about the size of a deck of cards. According to these recommendations, you can have a 3-ounce portion, four to six days per week or a 4-ounce portion three to four days per week. According to the American Heart Association, "It's OK to eat red meat, as long as you limit the amount. People should limit lean meat, skinless chicken, and non-fried fish to 5 ½ ounces per day, total." Additionally, in a recent review investigating the role of red meat in the Mediterranean diet, authors concluded, "Currently, there is not enough scientific evidence to suggest the strict limitation of the red meat consumption among the general population…" Again, the nutrition principle of **moderation** is important to implement when it comes to long-term health risk and disease prevention. Choosing fresh, unprocessed meats and limiting processed meats to once a week (i.e. deli meats, bacon, ham, and hot dogs) is another healthful way to incorporate meat into your meal plans.

DAIRY PRODUCTS

Dairy products include milk, yogurt, cheese, and kefir. As with meat, dairy products provide all nine essential amino acids and, therefore, are a significant source of high-quality protein. This is one of the remarkable differences between cow's milk and other "milks" or milk substitutes. While soy milk is similar in protein content to cow's milk, providing 8 grams per cup, almond, coconut, and rice milks have only 1 gram of protein per cup on average. Cow's milk is a nutrient-rich beverage, containing the following Daily Values in one cup:

Calcium - 30%

Phosphorus - 25%

Potassium - 10%

Riboflavin (vitamin B2) - 25%

Vitamin B12 - 20%

Vitamin A - 10%

Vitamin D - 25%.

The National Health and Nutrition Examination Survey (NHANES) is a program that collects health and nutrition data in order to identify the health needs of the United States and provide guidance on nation-wide health interventions. Unfortunately, NHANES data indicates fluid milk consumption decreases to just under 1 cup a day beginning at age 12, and only 48% of adolescents drink milk, which is a concerning food trend. Those who drink milk consume 180% more vitamin D and 49% more calcium than those who don't drink milk. Clearly, this is a substantial difference in nutrient intake among consumers versus non-consumers of milk.

The role of consuming dairy products for bone health is widely discussed because of their calcium, protein, phosphorus, and vitamin D content. However, there are additional health benefits beyond the prevention of osteoporosis. The Dietary Approach to Stop Hypertension (DASH) diet is promoted by the National Heart Lung and Blood Institute (NIH) as a healthy diet that is proven to lower blood pressure and reduce LDL cholesterol levels, the "bad" cholesterol contributing to heart disease if levels are too high. *U.S. News and World Report* also ranks the DASH diet, along with the Mediterranean Diet, as "Best Diet Overall" for health.

The DASH diet includes abundant servings of fruits, vegetables, and whole grains, along with nuts, lean protein, AND low-fat dairy products. This is because milk and dairy products are rich sources of calcium and potassium. Calcium impacts the contraction and relaxation of blood vessels, and several studies have shown diets higher in calcium have been related to lower blood-pressure levels. Potassium promotes urinary losses of sodium, resulting in a decrease in fluid retention and blood pressure. This combination of nutrients makes dairy an integral part of the DASH diet and an overall healthy, long-term diet approach.

Based on nutrient content, cheese (1 ½ ounces), yogurt (1 cup), and kefir (1 cup) can be used as alternatives for 1 cup of fluid milk. Hard cheeses, yogurt and kefir may be better tolerated by those with lactose intolerance, without having to fully omit dairy products from the diet. While kefir has grown in popularity and availability, based on my own experience with my clients, many have yet to try this fermented milk product. One of the strengths of kefir is the probiotic content. A recent review estimated that at least 300 microbial species are found in kefir, depending on the grain used during fermentation. Possible benefits attributed to kefir consumption include: anticancer effects, better blood-glucose control, as an anti-inflammatory, and reduction of blood pressure and cholesterol.

Stay tuned as more research is conducted on the health benefits of kefir. Yogurt, likewise, is a fermented dairy product, yielding probiotic content and associated health benefits. The benefits of consuming yogurt with active cultures include a healthy digestive system and a healthy immune system.

**Support the strength and structure of
your body with the power of protein.**

HOW TO EXPERIENCE THE POWER OF PROTEIN

- Grate some cheese and sprinkle over your soup or salad. Use soft, sharp and fresh cheeses to add flavor to almost any dish or combine with whole grain crackers or fruit for a delicious snack.

- Revisit your childhood with homemade macaroni and cheese. One of my favorite meals is macaroni and cheese with an almond crust. Instead of having this as your main dish, use it as a side dish, since the portion may be less overwhelming.

- Create a hamburger from a mix of ground meat and ground lentils or beans. Enjoy your half-veggie burger!

- Make it a taco-Tuesday-night with your protein of choice; this can include carne asada, carnitas, fish, or chicken. Top with salsa or tomatoes, cabbage, onions, and avocado for a balanced dinner option. If you are easily overwhelmed by portion sizes, make it street tacos for an even smaller size.

- Cook a hearty soup with meat (such as chicken noodle soup), a turkey and white bean chili, or a traditional stew.

- If you can hardly remember the last time you had a hamburger, start with a single slider—smaller than a standard sized hamburger. You can make them at home or choose them at a restaurant, since they are a common menu item.

- Try a cup of milk or yogurt in the morning as a part of a balanced breakfast including fruit and grains. If you make oatmeal, pour some of the milk into your oatmeal for added flavor and fluid.

- Sauté cubes of chicken breast with vegetables. This mixture can be incorporated into several different meal options, simply by changing the flavoring or sauce. For example, soy or teriyaki may be added during cooking as you create a stir fry with rice. Garlic sauce or tzatziki can be used, creating a Mediterranean-style dish with pita bread.

RECIPES

QUICK AND EASY TACO SOUP
SERVES 10-13

INGREDIENTS

1 pound ground beef

1 large onion, chopped

Garlic salt, to taste

3 (15 ounce) cans of beans of any of
the following: kidney beans,
black beans, chili-seasoned beans,
pinquinto beans, white beans or
pinto beans, or mixture of any of the

above

1 (15 ounce) can chopped tomatoes

1 (16 ounce) jar any kind of mild salsa

1 (16 ounce) Italian-style tomato sauce

½ c. fresh chopped cilantro

1 teaspoon cumin

Water (2 or 3 cups , based on desired
consistency)

TOPPING:

Grated cheddar cheese

Sour cream

Corn chips

Shredded lettuce

Chopped olives

INSTRUCTIONS

1. In large, deep pot, brown the beef and onion. Drain fat and season with garlic salt.

2. Add the canned beans, not drained, and the rest of the ingredients.

3. While the soup is simmering, prepare the toppings that will be added to each hot bowl of soup as desired.

Contributed by E.B.
Recipe from Cooking Something Up Cookbook

BACON WRAPPED DATES WITH GOAT CHEESE
SERVES 16

INGREDIENTS

8 slices bacon

16 dates

4 ounces goat cheese

Toothpicks

INSTRUCTIONS

1. Preheat oven to 350 degrees.

2. Slice dates lengthwise to create an opening. Remove the pit.

3. Put a small amount of goat cheese into each date and close by pressing the sides together.

4. Cut bacon slices in half. Wrap each date with a bacon slice and secure with a toothpick.

5. Arrange evenly on a baking sheet and bake for 10 minutes. Remove baking sheet and turn dates on their sides.

6. Bake for 5-8 more minutes, or until browned. Turn to other side and repeat.

7. Remove from oven and place on a plate lined with paper toweling and let cool.

Contributed by Katie Nili
Recipe adapted from Pinterest

INSTANT POT CHICKEN TACO BOWLS

SERVES 6

INGREDIENTS

1 cup low-sodium chicken broth

1 pound boneless skinless chicken breasts

1 packet taco seasoning

1 small, puréed onion

2 cloves garlic

15 ounces black beans (1 can), rinsed and drained

11 ounces canned corn

2 cups medium southwest salsa (key ingredient!!)

1/2 teaspoon cumin

1 cup rice, rinsed and drained

1/2 cup Mexican cheese to top

INSTRUCTIONS

1. Spray bottom of 6-quart Instant Pot (IP) with non-stick cooking spray.

2. Add 1/2 cup chicken broth to bottom of pot.

3. Add chicken breasts, taco seasoning, pureed onion and garlic cloves.

4. Add black beans, corn, salsa, cumin, rice and remaining 1/2 cup chicken broth.

5. Press rice into the liquid to make sure it's fully submerged.

6. Set valve to sealing. Cook on Manual (high pressure) for 8 minutes.

7. Allow pressure to naturally release for 12 minutes, then turn to quick release.

8. Remove IP lid and gently fluff rice with a fork (Don't stir it!).

9. Place IP lid back on (with power off) for 5 more minutes to allow rice to rest while you prepare the toppings.

10. Slide rice to the side a bit to find the chicken breasts and pull them out. Shred the chicken.

11. Add a scoop of rice mixture to a bowl. Top with some shredded chicken, and other desired toppings. Serve with tortillas, if desired.

Contributed by Samantha Lynes
Recipe adapted from TastesBetterfromScratch.com

POLLO ALLA CACCIATORA

SERVES 4-6

INGREDIENTS

1 (3 pound) chicken, cut into serving pieces, rinsed and patted dry

Salt and pepper

3 tablespoons olive oil

1 onion, sliced

1 large red bell pepper, cored, seeded, cut into thin strips

2 garlic cloves, minced

½ cup dry white wine

1 cup drained, peeled, and chopped tomatoes or 1 (28 oz) can peeled tomatoes, drained and chopped

1 teaspoon minced fresh oregano or ½ teaspoon dried oregano

1 teaspoon minced fresh thyme or ½ teaspoon dried thyme

1 bay leaf

2 tablespoons mince fresh basil leaves

INSTRUCTIONS

1. Season the chicken with salt and pepper.

2. In a large skillet over medium heat, cook the chicken in 2 tablespoons olive oil, turning occasionally, for 5-7 minutes, until browned. Transfer chicken to a plate.

3. Add 1 tablespoon olive oil and heat it until hot, coating skillet. Add onion, bell pepper, and garlic. Cook, stirring occasionally, for 5 minutes.

4. Add the wine and reduce for 1 minute.

5. Add tomatoes, oregano, thyme, bay leaf, salt and pepper, and bring mixture to a simmer.

6. Return chicken to skillet and simmer, covered, 25-30 minutes, until juices run clear. Transfer chicken to a serving platter.

7. Reduce the vegetable mixture in the skillet, stirring, until it is thick, about 3 minutes. Remove the bay leaf.

8. Spoon vegetable mixture over the chicken and sprinkle the dish with basil.

Contributed by Samantha Lynes
Recipe from The Best of Italy – a Cookbook by Evie Righter

BEAN AND TURKEY SAUSAGE STEW

SERVES 4

INGREDIENTS

1 tablespoon olive oil

1 (12 ounce) package fully cooked
smoked turkey sausage, sliced

2 cloves garlic, thinly sliced

1 (19 ounce) can cannellini beans, rinsed
and drained

1 (14.5 ounce) can low-sodium chicken
broth

1 (14.5 ounce) can diced tomatoes with
liquid

1 bunch spinach leaves, torn into 2-inch
pieces

Kosher salt and black pepper

1 ½ cups Tortellini

1 loaf country bread (optional)

INSTRUCTIONS

1. Heat the oil in a large saucepan or Dutch oven over medium heat. Add the sausage and cook, stirring once, until browned, 2 to 3 minutes.

2. Stir in the garlic and cook for 2 minutes more.

3. Add the beans, broth, and tomatoes. Bring to a boil.

4. Add the spinach and ¼ teaspoon each salt and pepper. Simmer, stirring occasionally, until wilted, 2 to 3 minutes.

5. Serve with the bread, if using.

Contributed by E.B.
Recipe adapted from realsimple.com by Anna Williams

SHEPHERD'S PIE
SERVES APPROXIMATELY 6

INGREDIENTS

1 pound lean ground beef

1 (1 ounce) envelope taco seasoning mix

¾ cup water

1 cup shredded cheddar cheese

1 (11 ounce) can whole kernel corn, drained

2 cups instant mashed potatoes, prepared

INSTRUCTIONS

1. Preheat oven at 350°F.

2. In skillet, brown beef, cook 10 minutes and drain.

3. Add taco seasoning and ¾ cup water. Cook for another 5 minutes.

4. Spoon beef mixture into 8-inch square baking pan. Sprinkle cheese on top.

5. Sprinkle with corn and spread mashed potatoes on top.

6. Bake for 25 minutes or until top is golden.

Contributed by Sydney Fox
Recipe from 1001 Easy Recipes Cookbook

FRENCH DIP SANDWICHES
SLOW-COOKER RECIPE
SERVES 8-10

INGREDIENTS

2 tablespoons olive oil

1 (2 ½ - 3 pound) beef roast (top and
bottom round roasts are preferable)

Kosher salt and freshly ground pepper

2 (1 ounce) packages dry onion soup mix

2 cups water

4 cups beef broth

8-10 crusty rolls or baguette thirds
(ciabatta rolls work great)

Swiss, provolone, or mozzarella,
shredded or sliced

INSTRUCTIONS

1. Heat 2 tablespoons of oil in large, high-sided pot or Dutch oven over medium high heat.

2. While oil is heating, season the roast on all sides with salt and pepper. Sear the roast on all sides, then transfer to the pot of a slow cooker.

3. Sprinkle with onion soup mix and add in water and beef broth.

4. Cook for 8-10 hours on low or start it on high (until it comes to a boil), then turn it to low and cook for another 4-5 hours on low. You'll know it's done when you pop a fork in it and the meat falls apart.

5. Cut rolls in half.

6. Shred the meat with two forks and place on crusty rolls.

7. Top with cheese and broil open face in the oven for 1-2 minutes or until the bread is golden and the cheese is melted.

8. Ladle au jus (the juices remaining in the cooker) into small cups for dipping and enjoy!

Contributed by E.B. "These are amazing!"
Recipe from ourbestbites.com by Kate Jones

5

THE ABILITY TO SAVOR SWEETS

Sweets, desserts, and sugary treats provide a sweetness to life and to food experiences. However, they are often associated with undisciplined eating choices, low willpower, and inevitable guilt that follows after indulging in them. Documentaries like "Fed Up" by Katie Couric haven't helped these perceptions, as it blames sugar for the weight issues of our society. You shouldn't feel guilty after consuming desserts and sweets. Why? Because eating them isn't wrong. You didn't commit a crime—you ate a cookie.

Julia Child said it well, "A party without cake is just a meeting." Sweet things should be celebratory, and a decadent dessert yields a sense of delight. Sweets and desserts are fun. They are tasty. They are pleasurable. And no one dessert will ruin your health-related goals, despite what you may project in your mind.

It's time to fully give yourself permission to eat sweets and desserts. No guilt. No shame. Time to get back to the party.

SEEKING PLEASURE IN FOOD

I commonly ask clients, "What value does food have?" I often get responses about vitamins, minerals, and physiological purposes. I quickly remind them about the value of taste and enjoyment. Indeed, studies indicate the major influencer of food decisions is taste. Seeking pleasure in food is an innate response and, yet, many try to dismiss it.

Research has shown that consuming foods high in sugar (and in fat) can increase endorphins (decreasing the feeling of stress) and can stimulate areas of the brain involved in reward and motivation. Your body and brain respond in a positive manner to the consumption of sweets. The relationship between sugar intake and reduction of stress is thought to be related to the hippocampus in the brain. Hippocampus activity includes regulation of emotions and creation of memories.

This is a fascinating piece of our physiology! Think of how many of your positive memories have a food-based component to them, as some food item is related to feelings of warmth and joy. Personally, when I eat a doughnut, I remember early Saturday mornings as a child, visiting yard sale after yard sale with my family. When I eat cake, I picture slathering my husband in frosting on our wedding day. Or, I can envision the years and years of frosting sugar cookies with my family during the Christmas season (trying to meticulously create the most beautiful version of each different shape). Some of you may be reading this but are associating desserts and sweets with poor memories or harsh experiences. I encourage you to seek help in this area, especially with a mental health expert, if you haven't done so already. Work to create positive experiences with these foods again.

Many cultures continue to promote pleasure in eating as an integral part of a healthy diet plan. Mark Singer, the technical director of cuisine at Le Cordon Bleu, says it well, "Food in France is still primarily about pleasure; cooking and eating are both pastime and pleasure." Italians also value savoring food. Meals are eaten slowly, as diners aim to derive pleasure during the eating experience and enjoy good company. And while seeking pleasure in food can be confused with unhealthy eating practices, research shows seeking pleasure leads to satisfaction. Satisfaction leads to the ability to stop eating or the prevention of overeating.

Here's how this typically plays out in sessions with my clients. They may crave ice cream, a food item that's sweet, has a smooth mouthfeel, and is cool to the tongue. Because of fear-based decision making or the perception that ice cream is a "bad" food, they choose a bag of carrots instead. The carrots fail to satisfy the craving. Next comes an apple. The apple also fails to satisfy, and next comes… Fairly soon, a trail of foods has been eaten, until they finally arrive at eating the ice cream, experienced with more intensity and greater feelings of guilt and failure. Seeking pleasure and satisfaction in your foods, along with achieving balance with your food options, allows you the freedom to choose sweets and desserts among the food choices you make on a daily basis.

ADDED VERSUS NATURAL SUGARS

Some people have started to confuse the difference between "added" and "natural sugars". Therefore,, they decide that it is best to eliminate ALL sugars from their diet. This is partly due to how food labels traditionally have provided the total sugar content of food and beverage products. (Note that this is set to change in 2020). Americans are frantically reading every food label and are stunned to note that sugar is in many products.

Carbohydrates are found in the form of monosaccharides (or single sugars), disaccharides (or two sugars), oligosaccharides and polysaccharides (multiple sugars chained together). Both mono- and disaccharides are considered simple sugars, and this is what you will find reflected on food labels under "Sugar". Simple sugars include glucose, fructose, galactose, maltose (produced during the fermentation of alcohol), sucrose (table sugar), and lactose (found in milk and dairy products). Dietary sources of sugar can include fruits, some vegetables, dairy products, and table sugar. Other sweeteners include honey, agave nectar, high fructose corn syrup, corn syrup solids, and molasses. Note that this list of sugar-containing foods includes fruits, vegetables, and dairy products—all significant sources of other essential nutrients along with glucose.

As you are exposed to comments from news and social media sources about how "bad" sugar is, keep in mind that these warnings are usually specific to "added" sugars. These are sugars that have been added to products during processing, cooking, or baking. I have met person after person who has eliminated certain fruits and vegetables from the diet to avoid the sugar content. If this is you, start reintroducing these items into your daily food plan. Fruits and vegetables contain fiber, phytochemicals, vitamins, and minerals—many beneficial compounds that promote health and energy. For example, I live in the Central Valley of California where small family strawberry farms and fruit stands populate many street corners. During the summer, the strawberries are abundant and are exceedingly sweet and delicious. That sweetness is due to the natural sugar content—8 grams of sugar per 8 medium strawberries. However, those strawberries provide 3 grams of dietary fiber, blunting the rise in blood sugar, along with potassium, folate, and more than the Daily Value for vitamin C.

This doesn't mean you should eat only fruits, vegetables, and dairy products, but then avoid all added sugars and prepared desserts. There is a distinct difference between the words "avoid" and "limit." "Limit" means added sugars CAN be a part of healthy diet.

HOW SWEETS FIT INTO A HEALTHY DIET

In the fall of 2010, Mark Haub, a nutrition professor at Kansas State University placed himself on the so-called "Twinkie Diet." It consisted mainly of eating Hostess Twinkies, powdered doughnuts, Little Debbie nutty bars, and similar packaged sweets every 3 hours. He limited his caloric intake each day and lost 27 pounds in a matter of 2 months. While this was a single case-study, the point is that the sweets and desserts did not promote weight gain. The treats were actually part of a weight loss plan. Additionally, blood markers for heart and metabolic disease improved. I'm not advocating this style of diet (nor was Mark). However, it lends to the understanding that SWEETS, IN AND OF THEMSELVES, ARE NOT SOLELY RESPONSIBLE FOR WEIGHT OR HEALTH ISSUES. They can be incorporated into a healthy diet. Similarly, the American Diabetes Association states: "Type 2 diabetes is not caused by sugar, but by genetics and lifestyle factors."

Integrating sweets and desserts into a healthy dietary plan may look different for different people. Some may have a strong "sweet tooth" and, therefore, enjoy them daily, while others find pleasure in desserts only during the weekend. It is partially determined by what you enjoy most and the prevalence of social circumstances when sweets become more available. An effective way to think about your added sugars is that they are a part of your daily discretionary calories. Discretionary calories are just that, you have the power to choose how you would like to use those calories.

Think of them as if they were part of your budget. You have an amount of money that must be used to meet your bills and essential needs, such as a mortgage or rent, food, gas, utilities, and insurance. Once these essentials have been covered, you may use any additional money for things like vacation, entertainment, and gifts. In the same way, you have a certain number of calories that you must consume to meet your base energy needs. Once you've consumed enough to provide your daily need for essential nutrients (vitamins, minerals, etc.), the rest of your calories can be used for "fun" (see the figure below). The nutritional value of these foods is not essential, and you may choose any food or beverage item simply for pleasure to meet your energy needs (i.e., sweets and desserts).

Recommendations for added sugars vary, depending on the health organization suggesting them. However, the theme is the same: Even though you shouldn't base your diet on added sugars, there is room for them in a healthy diet. Assuming you may be accustomed to establishing and following food "rules," note that recommendations surrounding added sugars are *guidelines*. That allows for more flexibility in your eating plan. The current Dietary Guidelines

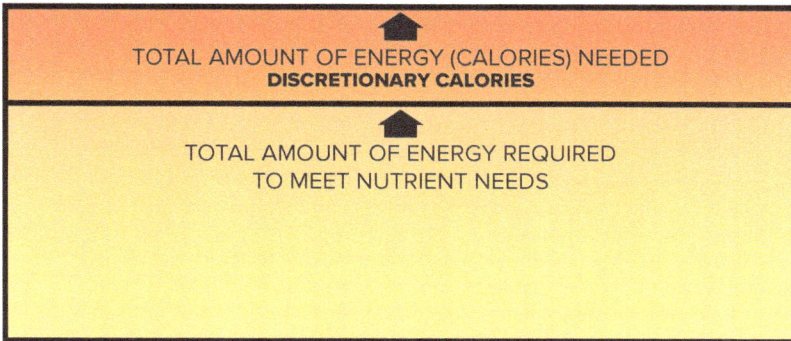

TOTAL AMOUNT OF ENERGY (CALORIES) NEEDED **DISCRETIONARY CALORIES**
TOTAL AMOUNT OF ENERGY REQUIRED **TO MEET NUTRIENT NEEDS**

Discretionary Calories

for Americans recommends limiting added sugars to no more than 10% of calories. Likewise, a 2018 statement by *American Family Physician* includes the recommendation to limit added sugars to no more than 5-10% of daily calories, consistent with recommendations by the World Health Organization. Again, these recommendations reflect research that shows EXCESSIVE intake of added sugars may yield negative health consequences, as compared to moderate consumption.

Once you have given yourself permission to include sugar in your diet, take the next step. Start by examining the sweets and desserts you derive the most pleasure from as you intentionally add them into your diet plan. Are you a chocolate lover? Someone who loves fruity flavors? Examine elements like texture and temperature. Are you more satisfied by a warm piece of apple pie or cold and creamy ice cream? How about a delicious combination of both as pie a la mode? Next, examine how you would fit desserts or treats into your day or week.

I've had clients who enjoy a sweet treat during the workday, since it promotes a sense of pleasure through the drudge of the day. Others like to end the day with the comfort of dessert. Still others I've worked with prefer to finish all lunches and dinners with a touch of something sweet, such as a square of chocolate. I recognize that the fear of sweets and desserts or a history of guilt may have disrupted your ability to identify what you truly enjoy. If this is you, it's time to experiment and commit to rediscovering what you love.

Reintroducing sugar into your diet may be a bite-by-bite process. Commit to one bite of a sweet treat first, then slowly add another bite at a different sitting until you're able to eat to a point of satisfaction. You may also want to mix sugary treats into more nutrient-dense food options as you challenge this area of your diet. For example, this may include adding whipped cream to a bowl of fruit, chocolate chips into trail mix, frozen yogurt into a smoothie, or chocolate syrup into milk. If you're working with a dietitian, discuss ideas with him or her.

SWEETS AND DISORDERED BEHAVIORS

I couldn't write this chapter on sweets without recognizing that you may avoid them because they have traditionally triggered disordered behaviors like bingeing and purging. Many of my clients haven't given themselves permission to eat them because they are afraid of losing control. If this describes you and/or you have used sweets as your main coping mechanism, that doesn't mean abstaining from sweets is a good long-term solution. Research substantiates this notion by the response of *counter-regulation.*

Counter-regulation refers to eating more of a food item than you would have expected to eat once you start eating it. This effect has been observed especially in the dieting and restricting populations, as opposed to those who don't engage in dieting or restrictive behaviors. For example, a study conducted at

Northwestern University investigated this response using milkshakes. Study subjects were given either zero, one, or two milkshakes as a "preload" and then were given access to as much ice cream as they desired. Those who identified themselves as dieters ate significantly more ice cream (despite drinking the milkshakes) than those who didn't diet. Basically, the dieters felt they had "blown" their diets and might as well continue eating without inhibition (counter-regulation), displaying an "all or nothing" mentality. Avoiding sweets promotes this counter-regulation effect. The experience of eating the sweets is done with great intensity.

Instead of avoidance, you can challenge yourself and strategize how to include sweets without engaging in a binge or overeating behavior. As identified earlier in this section, sweets promote reduction of stress and the release of dopamine, the "feel good" hormone. When my clients use sweets primarily for coping with emotions, the end result is usually guilt and shame. But, when they learn to seek pleasure in the eating experience and intentionally eat sweets, the end result is delight and satisfaction. If you've used sweets as your primary way of coping, it's time to identify new and effective coping mechanisms. Journaling, calling a friend, going for a walk, reading, listening to music, meditating, praying, breathing for 10 seconds, etc. The list of alternate coping behaviors is long. This can be an area to explore with a therapist as you work to discover what works uniquely for you.

Furthermore, if the presence of a sweet or dessert in the home consistently leads to a binge, it may be time to take another approach. Instead of having the ice cream in the house and finding lack of control, reintroduce it by going out for ice cream with others. Intentionally choose your favorite flavor. Once you feel calm with this decision, try bringing single-serve ice cream treats into the home, and be sure you consume these in the presence of others (as mentioned earlier, binges are often done in isolation). Be sure to strategize how to prevent a binge from happening, such as refraining from eating in your room. The eventual goal would be to achieve control AND pleasure from having your favorite bowl of ice cream in your home, being able to consume it mindfully and in moderation.

Whatever your history is with sweets, you can savor them again.

HOW TO SAVOR SWEETS

- Eat a small square of dark chocolate. Much research substantiates the health benefits of the cacao bean, which may help you take a small step in recognizing sweets as a part of a healthy diet.

- Eat a sweet at a social occasion when everyone else is eating them. It normalizes the behavior and can make it easier.

- Add fresh fruit or nuts to ice cream to create balance in your dessert item if you are having difficulty giving yourself permission for "fun" foods.

- Start with a nutrient-dense food item with added sugars such as a sweetened yogurt or sweetened cereal. (My husband's favorite is Cinnamon Toast Crunch).

- Bake with trusted friends or family members, committing to enjoy a piece of what you created. If it's a cake, pie, or dessert casserole, plate a small portion and taste it as a chef would, analyzing the quality of the creation.

- Try kettle corn, which combines the tastes of sweet and salty, along with a whole grain.

- Start with a single hard or chewy piece of candy. For example, caramel, a Tootsie Roll®, or a lemon drop.

- Purchase a kid-sized or mini ice cream. Gelato is often served in smaller cups, leading to less overwhelming servings.

RECIPES

ALMOND POPPY SEED BREAD
SERVES APPROXIMATELY 8

INGREDIENTS

3 cups all-purpose flour, lightly spooned into measuring cups and leveled with a knife

1 ½ teaspoons table salt

1 ½ teaspoons baking powder

3 eggs

1 cup + 2 tablespoons canola oil

2 ½ cups white sugar

1 ½ teaspoons vanilla extract

1 ½ teaspoons butter flavoring

1 ½ teaspoons almond flavoring

1 ½ cup milk or buttermilk

1 tablespoon poppy seeds

GLAZE:

¾ cup white granulated sugar

¼ cup orange juice

½ teaspoon vanilla

½ teaspoon butter flavoring

½ teaspoon almond flavoring

INSTRUCTIONS

1. Preheat oven to 350°F. Grease two standard-size bread pans or 5 mini bread pans. Set aside.
2. In a medium bowl, sift together flour, salt, and baking powder.
3. In a large mixing bowl, combine eggs, oil, sugar, extract and flavorings. Beat for 2 minutes.
4. Alternate adding in flour mixture and milk. Mix until just combined.
5. Add poppyseeds and mix until just combined.
6. Pour into prepared pans (5 mini pans or 2 standard bread pans), dividing equally, and bake (35-40 minutes for mini pans, 1 hour for large pans); keep an eye on them.
7. When done, place on a cooling rack and allow to cool completely.
8. While bread is cooling, prepare glaze by combining all glaze ingredients. Drizzle over loaves and allow to harden.

NOTE:

If possible, try not to package these in cellophane until ready to deliver (if you plan to bring to someone), because after a while, the moisture will condense in the bag and the glorious sugary crust on the bread will liquefy and soak into the bread. The bread will still taste great, but the slightly-crispy texture on top of the soft bread may just be the best part.

Contributed by E.B.
"They will definitely have this in Heaven!"
Recipe from ourbestbites.com by Kate Jones

BANANA BREAD

SERVES 1 LOAF OR APPROXIMATELY 10 SLICES

INGREDIENTS

¼ cup walnuts

3 bananas

½ cup butter

¾ cup sugar

3 eggs

2 cups flour

1 teaspoon baking soda

INSTRUCTIONS

1. Lightly grease a loaf pan and preheat oven to 375°F.

2. In a food processor, chop the nuts (coarsely chopped). Remove and set aside.

3. Cut the bananas into chunks and process in food processor until smooth. Scrape out work bowl and set aside.

4. Add the butter and sugar to food processor and process until creamy. Add eggs one at a time until blended. Add flour and baking soda. Process with ingredients in work bowl. Return bananas and nuts to work bowl and process until just blended.

5. Fill loaf pan. Bake for 52 minutes or until toothpick comes out clean.

6. Remove loaf from pan and cool for 15 minutes.

Contributed by Katie Nili

OATMEAL CARMELITAS

SERVES 36

INGREDIENTS

CRUST:

2 cups Pillsbury BEST® All Purpose or Unbleached Flour

2 cups quick-cooking rolled oats

1 ½ cups firmly packed brown sugar

1 teaspoon baking soda

½ teaspoon salt

1 ¼ cups margarine or butter, softened

FILLING:

1 (12.5 ounce) jar or 1 cup caramel ice cream topping

3 tablespoons Pillsbury BEST® All Purpose or Unbleached Flour

TOPPING:

1 (6 ounce) package or 1 cup semisweet chocolate chips

½ cup chopped nuts

INSTRUCTIONS

1. Heat oven to 350°F. Grease 13x9-inch pan.

2. Lightly spoon flour into measuring cup; level off with knife. In large bowl of a stand mixer, combine all crust ingredients; mix at low speed until crumbly. Reserve half of crumb mixture (about 3 cups) for topping. Press remaining crumb mixture in bottom of greased pan. Bake for 10 minutes.

3. Meanwhile, in a small bowl, prepare filling by combining caramel topping and 3 tablespoons flour; blend well with a spoon.

4. Remove partially baked crust from oven; sprinkle with chocolate chips and nuts. Drizzle evenly with caramel mixture; sprinkle with reserved crumb mixture.

5. Return to oven. Bake an additional 18 to 22 minutes or until golden brown. Cool 1 hour or until completely cooled. Refrigerate 1 to 2 hours or until filling is set. Cut into bars.

Contributed by Samantha Lynes
Recipe from Pillsbury.com

RAINBOW COOKIE BARS

SERVES APPROXIMATELY 16

INGREDIENTS

½ cup (1 stick) butter

2 cups graham crackers, crushed

1 (14 ounce) can sweetened condensed milk

⅔ cup flaked coconut

1 cup chopped pecans

1 cup M&M's

INSTRUCTIONS

1. Preheat oven to 350°F.

2. In 9 x 13-inch pan, melt butter in oven.

3. Sprinkle crumbs over butter and pour condensed milk over crumbs.

4. Top with coconut, pecans, and M&M's. Press down firmly.

5. Bake for 25-30 minutes or until light brown. Cool and cut into bars.

Contributed by Sydney Fox
Recipe from 1001 Easy Recipes Cookbook

SWEET POTATO CASSEROLE

SERVES 8

INGREDIENTS

2 pounds (about 3 large) sweet potatoes, peeled

⅓ cup unsalted butter, melted

½ cup light or dark brown sugar, packed

2 large eggs, beaten

½ cup heavy cream or whole milk

1 teaspoon pure vanilla extract

¼ teaspoon salt

TOPPING:

⅓ cup all-purpose flour

½ cup light or dark brown sugar, packed

½ teaspoon ground cinnamon

⅓ cup unsalted butter, melted

2 cups pecans

Optional: fresh rosemary or thyme, and sea salt for garnish, especially if using this as a side dish.

INSTRUCTIONS

1. Place the sweet potatoes in a large pot or Dutch oven. Add water to the pot until the potatoes are completely covered.

2. Cook on high until the water boils, then reduce heat and simmer for 20 minutes or until the potatoes are tender. Drain the cooked potatoes and allow them to cool for 15 minutes.

3. While potatoes are cooling, preheat the oven to 350°F. Grease a 9x13-inch baking pan or a 3-quart casserole dish.

4. Cut the potatoes into small chunks. Place them in a large mixing bowl or mixing bowl for a stand mixer. Beat the potatoes until smooth using a handheld or stand mixer. (You can create a really smooth consistency or leave it a little chunky.)

5. Mix in the butter, brown sugar, eggs, cream, vanilla extract, and salt. Pour the mixture into the greased pan or dish.

6. For the topping: Add the flour, brown sugar, and cinnamon to a medium bowl and whisk until well mixed. Carefully fold in the butter and pecans with a rubber spatula until the mixture is completely combined. Spread the mixture evenly over the potatoes with rubber spatula.

7. Place potatoes in the preheated oven and bake for 30-40 minutes or until topping looks golden brown. Allow dish to cool for 5 minutes and top with fresh rosemary and a touch of sea salt, if desired. This dish is best enjoyed warm.

MAKE AHEAD TIP:
This is a great make ahead recipe! You can prepare the potatoes through step 3 and refrigerate up to 2 days or freeze for up to 2 months.

NOTE:
While this isn't a traditional dessert, it's a fun side dish that incorporates added sugars with nutrient-rich sweet potatoes.

Contributed by Sydney Fox
Recipe from Sally McKenney of Sally's Baking Addiction

BRAZILIAN LEMONADE

SERVES 4

INGREDIENTS

6 cups cold water

1 cup sugar

4 juicy limes

6 tablespoons sweetened condensed milk

INSTRUCTIONS

1. Mix cold water and sugar very well and chill until ready to use. This step can be done ahead of time.

2. Wash limes thoroughly with soap (dishwashing soap or regular hand soap). Cut the ends off the limes and then cut each lime into 8ths.

3. Place ½ the limes in your blender.

4. Add ½ of the sugar water, place the lid on your blender and pulse 5 times. Place a fine mesh strainer over a pitcher and pour the blended mixture through the strainer and into the pitcher. Discard the pulp and other stuff in the strainer in the trash.

5. Repeat with remaining limes and sugar water.

6. Add sweetened condensed milk to the pitcher. Taste test at this point. If it comes out bitter, just add more sugar and maybe a little more milk.

7. Serve immediately over ice.

8. Note: This does not keep well, so do not make this in advance.

Contributed by E.B.
Recipe from ourbestbites.com by Sara Wells

6

THE DELIGHT OF DINING OUT

Virginia Woolf (English writer) said, "One cannot think well, love well, sleep well, if one has not dined well." Dining out can promote pleasure and enjoyment in foods. It provides new meal ideas, new ways to prepare food, new tastes, even introduces you to new cultures. It brings together family and friends in a shared event or experience. In his show, "Anthony Bourdain: Parts Unknown," the late Anthony Bourdain explored cultures around the globe. The conversations occur over shared meals as he learns about new locations and the traditions that define their people. This embodies the experience of dining out.

Too often, I encounter clients who demonstrate anxiety at the mention of dining out, instead of pleasure. When someone mentions meeting them at a restaurant, they experience immediate emotional distress, even to the point of panic. For others, dining out is done in secret, alone, and with shame. If you are one of these people, it's time to change your thinking about restaurant meals. As mentioned previously, one meal will not hinder your health-related goals. It's just one meal. Eating at restaurants is a part of normal eating behavior. You CAN dine well. The purpose of this chapter isn't to encourage dining at restaurants for every meal or even most of your meals. Instead, it's to encourage dining out in a manner that has health and social benefits, without a cloud of guilt, and without anxiety. Dining out should not be something you feel you need to compensate for (especially for those with disordered behaviors).

WHY EAT OUT?

In 2015, Americans spent just over $745 billion at restaurants. Twenty percent of Americans visit both full- and quick-service restaurants each week. Twenty-five percent of them purchase foods and beverages at coffee shops (Hello, Starbucks). Clearly, restaurant eating is a significant part of our American culture. The goal of healthy living isn't to avoid restaurants all together.

What is it about eating out that makes it such a large part of our American culture? One element is definitely the convenience. In this world of apps and automated ordering, it's fast and accessible for the busy family and busy working singles. Restaurants offer the value of time. Additionally, some people don't feel confident in their cooking skills, and find they enjoy the taste of food someone else has prepared. (I would love to see more culinary education in the school curriculum!)

Moreover, consumers eat out because of the dining experience at some restaurants. For children, the experience means getting to play in the play area (if the restaurant has one) while munching on some French fries. As we get older, we love being hosted, served, and taken care of as we sit with a nice meal and good company. Furthermore, we eat out simply to enjoy the taste. My husband and I traveled to New York and ate our way through the city, experiencing New York city bite-by-bite, savoring each new experience at each different restaurant.

Finally, we eat out to celebrate and come together with friends and family. No one has to cook. No one has to clean. Everyone gets to celebrate an accomplishment, a birthday, or any significant event (maybe simply making it through another week). The point is that there are many reasons to eat out that provide value to the consumer. I'm sure you can provide several more reasons through your own experience and exposure.

It's important to approach this area of nutrition with confidence and calm.

CREATING BALANCE

Creating a healthy eating out plan starts with frequency. As mentioned above, the goal of this chapter isn't to promote eating out every day, but to get you comfortable with the experience of eating out. If you are someone who eats at restaurants frequently due to job-related duties, then I know you have some specific challenges (such as constant exposure to larger portion sizes or "feeling heavy" from the food as my clients have complained about). I've worked with sales professionals who are either on the road throughout each day or must take clients out to meals for business discussions. If this is you, create balance by trying to consume homemade meals for those times when you aren't required to eat out for business.

If you are not required to eat out regularly and tend to avoid restaurants, challenge yourself to eat out approximately 1-2 times a week to start to acclimate yourself to the experience of restaurant dining. As you approach eating at restaurants, integrate the nutrition principle of moderation. (Truly, this is how you can approach everything in nutrition). Review your calendar and identify how to prioritize your restaurant meals. Do you have a night where you typically end the day later, and a restaurant meal would be helpful? Would a weekend dinner out with friends or family be a goal, providing necessary time to connect around a meal? Do you anticipate a day of travel and eating on the road?

MEAL CHOICE BALANCE

You can create balance in your meal choices while continuing to promote pleasure in your decision. To do so, let's revisit the basic food groups: grains, meat/beans, dairy, fruits and vegetables. Choose a meal that will cover 4 food groups to provide balance in your meal. For example, a chicken taco includes a grain (tortilla), meat/beans (chicken), vegetables (cabbage and salsa), and dairy (cheese). At a nice restaurant, it might be something like fish, chicken or steak, rice pilaf, side salad or grilled vegetables with cheese sprinkled on the salad. If you are at an event (such as a wedding or potluck) at which you plate your own food, divide your plate into thirds or quarters and place a different food group in each section. And don't forget about the value of fats. Be intentional about adding healthful fats like avocado, nuts, seeds, or a drizzle of oil to foods.

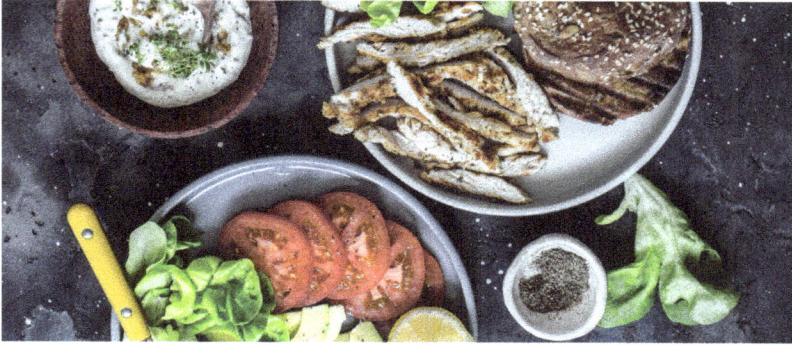

Example of a balanced meal

If you are working with a dietitian and following an individualized meal plan, that should be your guide to creating balance. If you are, however, eating intuitively (according to hunger and satiety cues) try to balance your food groups throughout the entire day. I have been to pancake breakfasts that offer pancakes, bacon, and coffee. That's it. I simply prioritize other food groups for later snacks and meals in order to create a balance of food groups. That might be choosing fruit as part of my snack or preparing a salad for my lunch. Or, if you are having a steak dinner one evening, meat may become less of a priority at lunch and, therefore, having a vegetarian style meal creates balance in your day.

However, creating balance does not mean restricting your food intake all day because you know you are having a larger, heartier dinner. It doesn't mean restricting your food intake the next day because you are afraid of weight gain associated with last night's dinner. Restricting is not a part of creating nutritional balance. Maintain a steady eating pattern.

**With these strategies in mind,
I'm hopeful you will reclaim
the delight of dining out.**

HOW TO REDUCE ANXIETY AT A RESTAURANT

When I worked in an intensive outpatient program several years ago, I remember feeling heartbroken over a particular patient who found it challenging to eat take-out. For 20 minutes, the patient sat and trembled in front of her chicken sandwich and French fries, only able to hold her French fry without eating a bite. The distress was palpable. I know the struggle is genuine for some of you. The following are steps for reducing anxiety when eating restaurant food, whether at the restaurant location or simply in another social eating situation, such as a barbeque, potluck, or wedding.

- Plan ahead. Take a look at the menu (without calorie counting) prior to attending the restaurant and choose your meal before you arrive. Tune into your taste buds, your thoughts, and feelings.

- Prepare visually for what you expect the meal will look like. If you believe the restaurant will be serving large portions, create a plan for how to manage the portion size to make it less overwhelming. Many of my clients will ask for a salad plate (a plate smaller than what dinner is being served on) so they can serve themselves how much they want on this smaller plate. It becomes less overwhelming. Or you might consider sharing your meal or a combination of appetizers to make a complete meal with protein, vegetables, and grains or starchy vegetables.

- Engage in conversation on topics that have nothing to do with food, diets, or weight. You will likely need to communicate this to others who are with you.

- Identify your goal before you eat the meal. For example, choosing what sounds satisfying versus what you perceive is the lightest meal on the menu, taking three bites of each food item, eating one plate of food at a potluck or buffet, or adding salad dressing to your salad. Goals can be significantly different; identify what feels doable for you.

- Be sure you are prepared with coping skills. Identify what normally works to provide "calm" for you. Maybe a stress ball, texting a friend, or eating outside with others where noise is minimal.

- Take your time. Take a deep breath and eat like a food critic. Notice taste, temperature, texture, and smell. It's okay to take a break from eating before returning to the meal.

- If you have an eating disorder (ED), identify what your eating disorder is telling you. Identify "truth" statements that combat the ED "voice." For example: ED speaking: "If you eat this meal you will gain 10 pounds." Truth: "One meal will not promote weight gain." Also, create a plan to abstain from any ED behaviors after the meal experience, whether you are vulnerable to bingeing, purging, or restricting. Communicate this plan to someone who will support you.

- Analyze how things went after the meal. What went well? What were the challenges? How can you do things differently next time? In their Intuitive

Eating worksheets, Evelyn Tribole and Elyse Resch term it "Learning and Letting Go." (Note: I highly recommend their book, *Intuitive Eating*.) It encourages you to see every eating experience as a learning experience versus labeling it with a "pass" or "fail." You are, then, better prepared for the next restaurant outing.

- Establish an "exit strategy." This is much easier done when attending a meal in someone's home or alternate venue, such as a wedding. If you feel overwhelmed, and panic is welling inside, an "exit strategy" may be stepping outside for a minute, going into someone's room (if you feel comfortable) with a trusted support person, or making a phone call in an alternate room to someone you know will encourage and calm you.

- Finally, if you only feel capable of eating small portions of the meal, you may want to have back up snacks, whether at home or with you on the go. You want to honor your hunger and nutrition needs.

7

THE ENJOYMENT OF EXERCISE

When I was in graduate school, I provided a nutrition talk to a 5th grade class. As I addressed nutrition and exercise, I asked the students, "If you exercise more, how does that change how much food you need?" The class answered unanimously and with great enthusiasm, "You need to eat less!" My heart sank. These 5th graders already associated exercise with weight loss goals. And why not? That's what we all hear about, right? Everyone is trying to exercise to promote weight loss; hence, eating less while exercising more. Exercise, then, becomes more about weight, and less about the multitude of benefits to be gained through regular physical activity.

Before I continue, I want to recognize that people reading this book are coming from a variety of experiences and attitudes about exercise.

- You are an athlete, and exercise means training with specific performance goals.

- You have an obsessive and destructive relationship with exercise. You are or have been compulsive with your exercise habits and are prone to over-exercising—seven days a week of exercising, doing sit-ups in the middle of the night, or engaging in more than one workout a day.

- You have been let down by exercise and demonstrate an "all or nothing" mindset with your exercise habits. If you don't lose 10 pounds in 2 weeks, exercise didn't deliver on its promise or meet your expectations. You then stop exercising, deciding the effort isn't worth the payoff.

- You may decide whether or not to exercise based on the number you see on the scale. If the number is "good," exercise doesn't matter. If the number is "bad," your gym bag is packed. The scale dictates your exercise pattern.

No matter your history with exercise, my goal is for you to implement exercise as a healthy part of your life-long plan. Not solely for weight control, but recognizing exercise as medicine for the mind and the body.

IMPORTANT NOTE: Any exercise plan must be approved by your doctor, team trainer, or treatment team. I would never recommend ignoring the advice of your medical team.

IT'S NOT SIMPLY ABOUT WEIGHT

According to the Centers for Disease Control (CDC), 47% of high school adolescents were trying to lose weight, based on the *Youth Risk Behavior Survey 2017*. Similarly, 49% of U.S. adults attempted to lose weight in a one-year period. As you would expect, exercise tops the list of strategies Americans incorporate to promote weight loss.

However, this limited focus on exercise yields negative consequences. It leads to obsessive desires about exercise for weight regulation and the perception that missing a day of exercise promotes weight gain in a single day. Many of my clients have attempted, on a day-by-day basis, to balance the calories **in** by *increasing* calories **out**. They will compensate for any additional calories by exercising more to "burn them off." For example, you'll find them rushing to the gym after a larger meal at a restaurant—to prevent what they perceive as inevitable weight gain.

Others start a regular exercise pattern for weight loss, and if results on the scale are not consistent with expectations, they stop. If exercise doesn't promote rapid weight loss, motivation for exercise plummets and the behavior stops (despite the amazing success of going from no exercise to four sessions of exercise a week!). Additionally, people at a healthy weight may naturally have low motivation for exercise because they don't need to lose weight.

Exercising for weight alone can encourage both excessive exercise and a sedentary lifestyle.

MENTAL HEALTH BENEFITS

When my husband is acting irritable, my usual response is to send him out the door to go for a run. His response is always, "I hate that you're right; exercise always makes me feel better." I appreciate how the authors of *Intuitive Eating* label their chapter on exercise, "Exercise—Feel the Difference." They write, "Shift your focus to how it feels to move your body, rather than the calorie-burning effect of exercise." Exercise feels good! It has a significant effect on stress-reduction, anxiety, depression, overall mood, and cognitive function.

MANAGING STRESS AND ANXIETY

Exercise promotes a range of physiological responses in the brain. This includes the release of norepinephrine in the areas of the brain involved in the body's emotional and stress response. *The increase of norepinephrine leads to an increase in motivation, working memory, and manages the actions of other neurotransmitters. This results in better management of stress and anxiety.*

However, scientists believe there is more to exercise and anxiety than a simple chemical explanation. Exercise provides an opportunity for the body to practice undergoing physical stress, but with positive outcomes. When you exercise, your heart rate increases, perspiration rate increases, and muscles are stimulated; the same physiologic response when you experience anxiety and stress. Jasper Smits, Ph.D. (Department of Psychology, Southern Methodist University, Dallas, Texas) and other study authors state it well in their study on the effect of exercise on anxiety: "Exercise, in many ways, is like exposure treatment. People learn to associate symptoms (the ones just mentioned—increased heart rate, etc.) with safety instead of danger." The communication pathways in the body get more efficient with repeated exposure, and situations that promote anxiety become easier to manage.

There is strong evidence that physical activity not only is effective at reducing symptoms for those experiencing anxiety in the moment, but also for those with anxiety disorders. No set recommended dose or duration of exercise has been identified to manage anxiety, whether acute or chronic. However, both resistance-exercise and aerobic-exercise have proven to be effective. This means you can utilize your preferred exercise method to help manage anxiety and stress.

DEALING WITH DEPRESSION

Likewise, research indicates that exercise is effective for treatment and prevention of depression. Indeed, many studies conclude that exercise is comparable to depression medications for patients with depressive disorders, and it can help to prevent relapse. In a 2013 systematic review, 83% of studies indicated that larger amounts of physical activity were effective for reducing risk of relapse.

If exercise is truly medicine for depression, then what amount seems to work? The good news is that moderate amounts, such as 20 minutes each day, have proven to be effective at reducing symptoms. However, studies have shown a dose-response relationship, with better outcomes resulting from more exercise. The Physical Activity Guidelines Advisory Committee (PAGAC) noted that there was a 48% risk reduction of depression from engaging in exercise more than 30 minutes per day. If you suffer from depression, your motivation to move may be extremely low for various reasons—fatigue, desire for isolation, and difficulty sleeping. You may need to recruit assistance and support from those you trust. It's encouraging to note that many studies will use moderate intensity activities, such as going for a brisk walk. You don't have to attend a high intensity gym workout, but simply walk out your door. See the figure below, for a list of moderate and vigorous intensity activities.

MODERATE-INTENSITY PHYSICAL ACTIVITY	VIGOROUS-INTENSITY PHYSICAL ACTIVITY
Brisk Walk	Running
Ballroom-Style Dancing	Aerobics
Bicycle (a pace of <10 miles/hour)	Bicycle (a pace of >10 miles/hour)
Water Aerobics	Heavy Construction Work
Doubles Tennis	Singles Tennis
Gardening	Jumping Rope

Examples of moderate and vigorous-intensity exercises

IMPROVING COGNITIVE FUNCTIONING

Finally, exercise is beneficial for cognitive functioning, including memory, learning, speed of processing information, and ability to focus. Engaging in a single session of moderate-to-intense exercise promotes these cognitive skills. This certainly encourages having P.E. classes in schools or taking a brisk walk at work to support the focus on essential tasks (with the added bonus of enhancing your mood!). While studies are mixed, approximately 10-20 minutes seems to be an optimal exercise duration to experience these benefits. Additionally, greater amounts of exercise have been effective for reducing risk with cognitive disorders like dementia and Alzheimer's. Recent research indicates risk reduction of cognitive decline by approximately 38-40% among those who regularly engage in physical activity. The Alzheimer's Association states, "Regular physical exercise may be a beneficial strategy to lower the risk of Alzheimer's and vascular dementia. Exercise may directly benefit brain cells by increasing blood and oxygen flow in the brain." Exercise has been shown to impact other markers of brain health, including volume and connectivity within the brain, as well.

Exercise is medicine for the mind and for your mood.

MEDICAL BENEFITS

The health benefits of exercise are numerous—truly impossible to cover in this small section! However, it's important to understand how exercise positively impacts chronic disease risk, without a specific focus on weight loss. Exercise plays a preventive role in: several cancers including breast cancer and colorectal cancer, bone health, type II diabetes, all-cause mortality (risk of death), heart disease, hypertension, stroke, and it can promote productive sleep. Recently, I was attending a doctor's appointment with my husband, and was elated when he wrote "exercise" on the prescription pad. He wanted to ensure that my husband knew exercise continued to be a part of his treatment plan. Exercise is medicine for the body.

Many studies have investigated the relationship between exercise and all-cause mortality. According to the 2018 Physical Activity Guidelines Advisory Committee (PAGAC) Scientific Report, benefits of exercise on all-cause mortality start with the lowest level of exercise—if you engage in any level of regular physical activity, you may reduce your risk of death. Hopefully, this evidence challenges any perfectionist tendencies you possess around exercise. Seventy percent of the potential benefit is reached by engaging in 150 minutes of moderate to vigorous activity each week. This equates to 30 minutes a day if you are active 5 days a week. This impacts those who have already been diagnosed with a chronic disease, including those with type II diabetes. A position paper released by the European Association of Preventive Cardiology 2019 recommends that those with type II diabetes should engage in 3-5 sessions of exercise per week to reduce mortality risk, especially because of associated improvements in blood sugar control. This recommendation was made without regard to body mass index as a specific target. Likewise, physical activity was shown to reduce risk of death from cardiovascular disease even from just simply walking.

When you exercise, the demand for delivery of oxygen to the muscles increases. Therefore, the heart pumps a greater volume of blood at a faster rate to meet the need. With greater training and exercise, the volume of blood pumped by the left ventricle of the heart (called the stroke volume) gets larger, and the heart essentially becomes more efficient. Regular exercise also increases the diameter of the blood vessels, resulting in lower resting blood pressure and lower resting heart rate. Exercise also results in adaptations in the muscles; it improves their ability to pull oxygen from the blood, reducing the workload of the heart muscle.

The list of positive benefits is long. And while heart disease continues to be the leading cause of death in the U.S., exercise is certainly a part of the prescription for change. According to a recent review, achieving 150 minutes of moderate intensity activity reduced risk of cardiovascular disease by 17% and death related to cardiovascular disease by 23%. Authors noted that the greatest reduction of risk occurred when subjects changed from low- to moderate-intensity exercise, more so than those who changed from moderate- to high-intensity exercise. Furthermore, they stated that their results suggest that "the majority of the health benefit that accrues from increasing PA (physical activity) is mediated by mechanisms beyond weight maintenance." To sum it up, your heart benefits from exercise without having to engage in highly intense exercise and without serious reductions in the number on the scale.

Furthermore, exercise is recommended in the fight against and prevention of several cancers. Evidence supports reduction in the risk of bladder cancer, breast cancer, colon cancer, endometrial cancer (lining of the uterus), adenocarcinoma of the esophagus, gastric cancer (stomach), renal cancer (kidneys), and lung cancer. Many of these are the more common cancers diagnosed in the U.S. According to the American Cancer Society, about 40% of men and about 38% of women are at risk of developing some kind of cancer—approximately 1 in every 3 people. They recommend at least 150 minutes of moderate-intensity exercise (or 75 minutes of vigorous-intensity exercise) each week for cancer prevention. They also state, "Doing some physical activity above usual activities, no matter what one's level of activity, can have many health benefits." Again, movement matters, and it doesn't require a rigid 2 hours a day in the gym to promote cancer prevention.

If you are someone who has engaged in compulsive or excessive exercise, note that you may put yourself at a **greater** health risk by continuing that trend. While a host of benefits are listed above, it's important to note that those recommendations are provided within the context of medical appropriateness. Exercising against medical advice may lead to cardiac arrest, injury to the muscle, loss of menstrual cycle, fatigue, bone density loss, dehydration and electrolyte imbalance, and increased incidence of illness and respiratory infection. If this is you, the heathiest step is to first seek help for managing your exercise behavior.

Additionally, you place yourself at risk if you engage in excessive exercise in a nutritionally compromised state without adequate energy intake and appropriate nutrition recovery practices. Refer to the RED-S state as discussed in the first chapter of this book. It is worth repeating here. Low energy availability contributes to poor sports performance and medical consequences. It leads to both loss of fat mass AND loss of lean body mass (which includes muscle mass and bone tissue). Many of my clients mistakenly believe that calorie restriction, combined with high levels of exercise, leads to a loss of body fat alone. However, the body will break down lean body mass as you place it under a high amount of stress without adequate rest and nutrition recovery. High school athletes engaging in disordered eating are twice as likely to suffer from a musculoskeletal injury, such as stress fractures and ligament sprains. Furthermore, overtraining syndrome, or burnout, is a condition perpetuated by both physical and mental stress. Athletes experience declining performance, despite training efforts, and face frequent injuries, infections, and changes in mood. Whether you are a serious athlete or every day exerciser, you are risking injury, disease and death by stressing your body without adequate fuel and nutrients.

Return to the enjoyment of exercise and gain appreciation for all your body is capable of.

HOW TO CREATE YOUR PLAN

When creating an exercise plan, there are many things to consider, such as previous experience with exercise, what you enjoy, what you can afford, what your body will benefit from, family/school/work life, scheduling needs, and possible physical limitations. You may have a training plan already structured for you because of participation in sports, which simplifies this process. However, you may be moving from high school, college, or elite competition into creating an exercise plan on your own. Wherever you place yourself now, keep in mind that an exercise plan will often require some flexibility. Circumstances change, and it's important to be able to roll with the inevitable transitions in life.

As the hip-hop recording artist and rapper L.L. Cool J said, "When you have a clear vision of your goal, it's easier to take the first step toward it." Here are steps for moving forward:

- Start with a conversation with your doctor, medical, or treatment team. Discuss any physical or medical concerns.

- Utilize fitness and exercise professionals who know what they are talking about and are appropriately trained/certified. This includes physical therapists and personal trainers certified by one of the following: National Strength and Conditioning Association (NSCA) with a Certified Strength and Conditioning Specialist (CSCS) certification, American Council on Exercise (ACE), American College of Sports Medicine (ACSM), and Exercise Physiologist (EP-C).

- Identify your current fitness level. Are you a trained athlete or someone who hasn't engaged in exercise in several years? If you haven't participated in an exercise program for a while, start slowly and with lower intensity. Walking is a great place to begin. You can always build from there. But high-intensity fitness is likely not going to be your best place to start (and is a great way to get injured!).

- When were you most successful with an exercise plan? Identify what you were doing then and what made it work. For example, you participated in a walk/run club and the structure and accountability promoted consistency and enjoyment.

- What does your budget allow for? You may love the idea of going to a small studio but those can be more costly. The value of signing up can absolutely be worth it, but not if it creates financial strain.

- What types of exercise sound more appealing? What brings you joy? Are you inspired by loud music at an aerobics class or do you love the peacefulness and quiet of yoga?

- Create a balanced exercise plan. Be sure to include cardiovascular workouts and strength and resistance training in your plan...with plenty of stretching! At least 150 minutes of cardiovascular work is recommended and at least two sessions of strength/resistance training each week. Resistance and weight training promote balance, strength, appropriate posture and bone health. Spending limitless hours on the treadmill or elliptical is not a healthy or balanced plan.

- Do you have a specific goal you can implement, such as completing a more strenuous hike or participating in a race? Some of my clients have had great success adding these types of events into their exercise plan, since it shifts the focus of exercise from weight to achievement.

- Add your exercise plan to your weekly calendar. Make it an appointment for yourself, just as if you were headed to a doctor's appointment.

- If you tend to be TOO rigid with your exercise plan, work on flexibility. I have my clients write one workout each on small pieces of paper, including one with the words "No Exercise", and place them all into a hat (or some kind of container). They then pull one piece of paper from the hat and do whatever is indicated that day. We create a variety of options, including different workout durations and types of exercise. For example, "45 minutes of yoga" or "one aerobics class." You need to be completely honest with this system. When you pull out one piece of paper, don't put it back. When you've gone through all the exercise options, put them all back into the container and start again.

- Identify whether you prefer to work out alone or with others. Is the accountability and support provided in social situations more desirable? Do you like to go into the great outdoors, put headphones on, and tune out from the rest of the world? At our office, we often use the phrase, "Find your fitness soulmate." Most people are more successful when they have someone to participate with them in workouts. It can also provide accountability if you tend to be too compulsive or rigid with your workouts.

REFERENCES

CHAPTER ONE

1. "Morbidity and Mortality Weekly Report: QuickStats: Percentage of Adults Who Often Felt Very Tired or Exhausted in the Past 3 Months, by Sex and Age Group" - National Health Interview Survey, United States, 2010-2011. Centers for Disease Control and Prevention. https://www.cdc.gov/mmwr/preview/mmwrhtml/mm6214a5.htm

2. Consumer Reports, 2017. "Tired and Low on Energy: Here are Some Nondrug Remedies". The Washington Post, 2017. https://www.washingtonpost.com/national/health-science/tired-and-low-on-energy-here-are-some-nondrug-remedies/2017/05/12/9aecada0-0e5b-11e7-9b0d-d27c98455440_story.html?noredirect=on&utm_term=.0d426f5b4676

3. "Energy Drinks Market Analysis By Product (Alcoholic, Non-Alcoholic), Product Type (Non-Organic, Organic, Natural), Target Consumer (Teenagers, Adults, Geriatric), Distribution Channel (On-Trade, Off-Trade & Direct Selling) And Segment Forecasts, 2018-2025". Grand View Research, 2017. https://www.grandviewresearch.com/industry-analysis/energy-drinks-market

4. Betts, JG, DeSaix, P, Johnson, E, Johnson, JE, Korol, O, Kruse, DH, Poe,B, Wise, JA, and Young, KA. 2018. Anatomy and Physiology: The Small and Large Intestines. OpenStax College. https://opentextbc.ca/anatomyandphysiology/chapter/23-5-the-small-and-large-intestines/

5. Müller, MJ, Enderle, Pourhassan, M, Braun, W, Eggeling, B, Lagerpusch, M, Glüer, CC, Kehayias, JJ, Kiosz, D, and Bosy-Westphal, A. 2015. "Metabolic adaptation to caloric restriction and subsequent refeeding: the Minnesota Starvation Experiment revisited". Am J Clin Nutr 102: 807-819.

6. Mattar, L, Huas, C, Duclos, J, Apfel, A, and Godart, N. 2011. "Relationship between malnutrition and depression or anxiety in Anorexia Nervosa: a critical review of the literature". J Affect Disord 132: 311-318.

7. Gauthier, C, Hassler, C, Mattar, L, Launay, JM, Callebert, J, Steiger, H, Melchior, JC, Falissard, B, Berthoz, S, Mourier-Soleillant, V, Lang, F, Delorme, M, Pommereau, X, Gerardin, P, Bioulac, S, Bouvard, M; EVHAN Group, Godart, N. 2014. "Symptoms of depression and anxiety in anorexia nervosa: Links with plasma tryptophan and serotonin metabolism".

Psychoneuroendocrinology 39: 170-178.

8. Superior Mesenteric Artery Syndrome. NIH: Genetic and Rare Diseases Information Center.
    https://rarediseases.info.nih.gov/diseases/7712/superior-mesenteric-artery-syndrome

9. Nattiv, A, Loucks, AB, Manore, MM, Sanborn, CF, Sungot-Borgen, J, and Warren, MP. 2007.
    "American College of Sports Medicine Position Stand: The Female Athlete Triad". Official
    Journal of the American College of Sports Medicine 39:1867-1882.

10. Mountjoy, M, Sundgot-Borgen, J, Burke, L, Carter, S, Constantini, N, Lebrun, C, Meyer,
    N, Sherman, R, Steffen, K, Budgett, R, and Ljungqvist, A. 2014. "The IOC consensus
    statement: beyond the Female Athlete Triad–Relative Energy Deficiency in Sport (RED-
    S)". British Journal of Sports Medicine 48: 491-497.

11. Shepphird, SF. 2011. Athletes and Anorexia Nervosa: An Elite Athlete's Story.
    http://www.drshepp.com/athletes-and-anorexia-nervosa-an-elite-athletes-story/

CHAPTER TWO

1. Whole Grains 101. Oldways Whole Grain Council. www.wholegrainscouncil.org

2. All About the Grains Group. United States Department of Agriculture. www.choosemyplate.
    gov

3. U.S.D.A. Food Composition Database: https://ndb.nal.usda.gov/ndb/

4. Mergenthaler, P, Lindauer, U, Dienel, GA, and Meisel, A. 2013. "Sugar for the Brain: The
    Role of Glucose in Physiological and Pathological Brain Function". Trends Neurosci. 36:
    587–597.

5. Croll, PH, Voortman, T, Ikram, MA, Franco, OH, Schoufour, JD, Bos, D, and Vernooij, MW.
    2018. "Better diet quality relates to larger brain tissue volumes: The Rotterdam Study".
    Neurology 90: e2166-e2173.

6. Jacobs Jr., DR, Andersen, LF, and Blomhoff, R. "Whole-grain Consumption is Associated
    with a Reduced Risk of Noncardiovascular, Noncancer Death Attributed to Inflammatory
    Diseases in the Iowa Women's Health Study". The American Journal of Clinical Nutrition
    85: 1606–1614.

7. Freedom Foods Group Limited. "Fiber is More than Just Roughage: The Emerging Role of
    Prebiotics on Gut Health". Today's Dietitian Symposium. Presented May 21, 2018.

8. Weight Management Dietetic Practice Group. "Modulating the GI Microbiome: Using Key
    Dietary Nutrients". Webinar Presented by Heiman, ML and Doyle, M. March 1, 2018.

CHAPTER 3

1. Vitamins. The Linus Pauling Institute: Micronutrient Information Center. Oregon State University. https://lpi.oregonstate.edu/mic/vitamins. This link leads to a website provided by the Linus Pauling Institute at Oregon State University. Sunny Yingling is not affiliated or endorsed by the Linus Pauling Institute or Oregon State University.

2. Platel, C, Cooper, D, Papadimitriou, JM, and Hall, JC. 2000. "The Omentum". World J Gastroenterol 6: 169–176.

3. Guerre-Millo, M. 2002. "Adipose Tissue Hormones". Journal of Endocrinological Investigation 25: 855-861.

4. Chang, CY, Ke, DS and Chen, JY. 2009. "Essential fatty acids and human brain". Acta Neurol Taiwan 18:231-241.

5. Essential Fatty Acids. The Linus Pauling Institute: Micronutrient Information Center. Oregon State University. https://lpi.oregonstate.edu/mic/other-nutrients/essential-fatty-acids #membrane-structure-function. This link leads to a website provided by the Linus Pauling Institute at Oregon State University. Sunny Yingling is not affiliated or endorsed by the Linus Pauling Institute or Oregon State University.

6. Kaiser, LL, Campbell, CG, and Academy Positions Committee Workgroup. 2014. Practice Paper of the Academy of Nutrition and Dietetics: Nutrition for a Healthy Pregnancy Outcome. J Acad of Nutr and Diet 114: 1447.

7. Tanaka, K, Farooqui, AA, Siddiqi, NJ, Alhomida, AS, and Ong, W-Y. 2012. "Effects of Docosahexaenoic Acid on Neurotransmission". Biomol Ther (Seoul) 20: 152-157.

8. Fish and Omega-3 Fatty Acids. Last Reviewed March 23, 2017. The American Heart Association. https://www.heart.org/en/healthy-living/healthy-eating/eat-smart/fats/fish-and-omega-3-fatty-acids

9. San Jose State University, NUFS 101 A/B: Food Science. Instruction and Materials by Perry, M.

CHAPTER 4

1. Ophardt, CE. 2003. Virtual Chembook: Overview of Protein Metabolism. Elmhurst College. http://chemistry.elmhurst.edu/vchembook/630proteinmet.html

2. U.S.D.A. Food Composition Database: https://ndb.nal.usda.gov/ndb/

3. Greenblatt, J and Delane, D. 2018. "Zinc Supplementation in Anorexia Nervosa". Journal of Orthomolecular Medicine 33(1)

4. Zelman, K. 2017. "Micronutrients: Choline". Food and Nutrition Magazine.

https://foodandnutrition.org/from-the-magazine/micronutrients-choline/

5. Burd, NA and Phillips, SM. 2017. Sports Nutrition: A Handbook for Professionals (6th edition). "Protein and Exercise". Chicago: Academy of Nutrition and Dietetics, 2017.

6. "Diet, Nutrition, Physical Activity and Cancer: A global Perspective". Continuous Update Project Expert Report 2018. World Cancer Research Fund/American Institute for Cancer Research.

    http://www.aicr.org/reduce-your-cancer-risk/recommendations-for-cancer-prevention/

7. Uzhova, I and Peñalvo, JL. 2018. "Mediterranean Diet and Cardio-metabolic Health: What is the Role of Meat?" Eur J Clin Nutr. 72:4-7.

8. National Dairy Council: Milk Comparison Chart. Originally published March 17, 2015.

    https://www.nationaldairycouncil.org/content/2015/whats-in-your-glass-infographic

9. Sebastian, RS, Goldman, JD, Wilkinson Enns, C; and LaComb, RP. 2010. "Fluid Milk Consumption in the United States: What We Eat In America", NHANES 2005-2006.

    https://www.ars.usda.gov/ARSUserFiles/80400530/pdf/DBrief/3_milk_consumption_0506.pdf

10. High Blood Pressure. The Linus Pauling Institute: Micronutrient Information Center. Oregon State University.

    https://lpi.oregonstate.edu/mic/health-disease/high-blood-pressure. This link leads to a website provided by the Linus Pauling Institute at Oregon State University. Sunny Yingling is not affiliated or endorsed by the Linus Pauling Institute or Oregon State University.

CHAPTER 5

1. The Determinants of Food Choice. 2006. The European Food Information Council.

    https://www.eufic.org/en/healthy-living/article/the-determinants-of-food-choice

2. Low, E. 2015. "Ask the Brain: Why Do We Crave Sugar When We're Stressed?" SITN Boston: Harvard University.

    http://sitn.hms.harvard.edu/flash/2015/ask-the-brain-why-do-we-crave-sugar-when-were-stressed/

3. "Memory, Learning, and Emotion: the Hippocampus". Updated 2014. Psycheducation.org.

    http://psycheducation.org/brain-tours/memory-learning-and-emotion-the-hippocampus/

4. Choi, AS. 2014. "What Americans Can Learn from Other Food Cultures". TED.

    https://ideas.ted.com/what-americans-can-learn-from-other-food-cultures/

5. Health Professionals: Toolkits. The California Strawberry Commission.

http://www.calstrawberry.com/en-us/Nutrition/Health-Professionals

6. Park, M. 2010. "Twinkie Diet Helps Nutrition Professor Lose 27 Pounds". CNN.

http://www.cnn.com/2010/HEALTH/11/08/twinkie.diet.professor/index.html

7. Diabetes Myths. Last edited August 20, 2018. American Diabetes Association.

http://www.diabetes.org/diabetes-basics/myths/?loc=db-slabnav

8. Sugar 101: Last Reviewed April 17, 2018. The American Heart Association.

https://www.heart.org/en/healthy-living/healthy-eating/eat-smart/sugar/sugar-101

9. Locke, A, Schneiderhan, J, and Zick, SM. 2018. "Diets for Health: Goals and Guidelines". Am Fam Physician 97: 721-728.

10. "Counterregulation of Eating". Psychology.

https://psychology.iresearchnet.com/social-psychology/antisocial-behavior/counterregulation-of-eating/

CHAPTER 6

1. "Eating out behavior in the U.S. - Statistics & Facts". Statista: The Statistics Portal.

https://www.statista.com/topics/1957/eating-out-behavior-in-the-us/ [Accessed January 2, 2019]

2. Millen, B, Lichtenstein, AH, Abrams, S, Adams-Campbell, L, Anderson, C, Brenna, JT, Campbell, W, Clinton, S, Foster, G, Hu, F, Nelson, M, Neuhouser, M, Perez-Escamilla, R, Siega-Riz, AM, and Story, M. 2015. USDA Scientific Report of the 2015 Dietary Guidelines Advisory Committee. https://ods.od.nih.gov/pubs/2015_DGAC_Scientific_Report.pdf

3. Setnick, J. 2017. Academy of Nutrition and Dietetics Pocket Guide to Eating Disorders (2nd edition). Chicago: Academy of Nutrition and Dietetics, 2017.

4. 9 Tips for Eating Out at Restaurants While in Eating Disorder Recovery. Eating Recovery Center.

https://www.eatingrecoverycenter.com/families/portal/meal-management/9-tips-for-eating-out-at-restaurants-while-in-eating-disorder-recovery [Accessed January 9, 2019.]

5. Tribole, E. and Resch, E. 2012. Intuitive Eating: A Revolutionary Program that Works. New York: St. Martin's Griffin, 2012.

CHAPTER 7

1. Kann, L; McManus, T; Harris, WA, Shanklin, SL; Flint, KH; Queen, B; Lowry, R; Chyen,

D; Whittle, L; Thornton, J; Lim, C; Bradford, D; Yamakawa, Y; Leon, M; Brener, N, and Ethier, KA. "Youth Risk Behavior Surveillance—United States, 2017". June 15, 2018. Center for Disease Control and Prevention Morbidity and Mortality Weekly Report. https://www.cdc.gov/healthyyouth/data/yrbs/pdf/2017/ss6708.pdf

2. Martin, CB, Herrick, KA, Sarafrazi, N, and Ogden, CL. 2018. Attempts to Lose Weight Among Adults in the United States, 2013–2016. Centers for Disease Control and Prevention National Center for Health Statistics. https://www.cdc.gov/nchs/products/databriefs/db313.htm

3. Tribole, E. and Resch, E. 2012. Intuitive Eating: A Revolutionary Program that Works. New York: St. Martin's Griffin, 2012.

4. Physical Activity Guidelines Advisory Committee Scientific Report: 2018. Office of Disease Prevention and Health Promotion. https://health.gov/paguidelines/second-edition/report/

5. Exercise fuels the brain's stress buffers. American Psychological Association. https://www.apa.org/helpcenter/exercise-stress.aspx [Accessed January 16, 2019]

6. Smits, JAJ, Berry, AC, Rosenfield, D, Powers, MB, Behar, E, and Otto, MW. 2008. "Reducing anxiety sensitivity with exercise". Depression and Anxiety 25: 689-699.

7. Wurtman, JJ. 2018. "Might Physical Activity be as Effective as Antidepressants?" Psychology Today. https://www.psychologytoday.com/ca/blog/the-antidepressant-diet/201811/might-physical-activity-be-effective-antidepressants

8. Kemps, H, Krankel, N, Dorr, M, Moholdt, T, Wilhelm, M, Paneni, F, Serratosa, L, Solberg, EE, Hansen, D, Halle, M, and Guazzi, M. 2019. "Exercise Training for Patients with Type 2 Diabetes and Cardiovascular Disease: What to Pursue and How to Do It". A Position Paper of the European Association of Preventive Cardiology (EAPC). European Journal of Preventative Cardiology 0: 1-19.

9. Wahid, A, Manek, N, Nichols, M, Kelly, P, Foster, C, Webster, P, Kaur, A, Friedemann Smith, C, Wilkins, E, Rayner, M, PhD, Roberts, N, and Scarborough, P. 2016. "Quantifying the Association Between Physical Activity and Cardiovascular Disease and Diabetes: A Systematic Review and Meta-Analysis. J Am Heart Assoc 5: e002495.

10. Summary of the ACS Guidelines on Nutrition and Physical Activity. Last Revised February 2016. American Cancer Society. https://www.cancer.org/healthy/eat-healthy-get-active/acs-guidelines-nutrition-physical-

activity-cancer-prevention/summary.html

11. Scotti, A. 2018. "25 Fitness Quotes to Push You Through Your Toughest Workouts". Men's Health.
    https://www.menshealth.com/fitness/a19547200/best-fitness-quotes-of-all-time/

12. Mayo Clinic Staff. 2018. Fitness: Create a Program that's Right for You. Mayo Foundation for Medical Education and Research
    https://www.mayoclinic.org/healthy-lifestyle/fitness/in-depth/fitness/art-20044002

www.ingramcontent.com/pod-product-compliance
Lightning Source LLC
Chambersburg PA
CBHW040927210326
41597CB00030B/5205